BREAK THE PATTERN OF

Yo-Yo

DIETING FOREVER!

Also by Doreen Virtue

Books/Kits/Oracle Board

ANGEL NUMBERS 101 (available July 2008)
SOLOMON'S ANGELS (a novel)
ANGEL BLESSINGS CANDLE KIT (includes booklet, CD, journal, etc.)
THANK YOU, ANGELS! (children's book with Kristina Tracy)
HEALING WORDS FROM THE ANGELS
HOW TO HEAR YOUR ANGELS
REALMS OF THE EARTH ANGELS
FAIRIES 101
DAILY GUIDANCE FROM YOUR ANGELS
DIVINE MAGIC
HOW TO GIVE AN ANGEL CARD READING KIT
ANGELS 101
ANGEL GUIDANCE BOARD
GODDESSES & ANGELS
CRYSTAL THERAPY (with Judith Lukomski)
CONNECTING WITH YOUR ANGELS KIT (includes booklet, CD, journal, etc.)
ANGEL MEDICINE
THE CRYSTAL CHILDREN
ARCHANGELS & ASCENDED MASTERS
EARTH ANGELS
MESSAGES FROM YOUR ANGELS
ANGEL VISIONS II
EATING IN THE LIGHT (with Becky Prelitz, MFT, RD)
THE CARE AND FEEDING OF INDIGO CHILDREN
HEALING WITH THE FAIRIES
ANGEL VISIONS
DIVINE PRESCRIPTIONS
HEALING WITH THE ANGELS
"I'D CHANGE MY LIFE IF I HAD MORE TIME"
DIVINE GUIDANCE
CHAKRA CLEARING (available in tradepaper, and as a hardcover book-with-CD)
ANGEL THERAPY®
THE LIGHTWORKER'S WAY
CONSTANT CRAVING A–Z
CONSTANT CRAVING

Audio/CD Programmes

ANGEL THERAPY® MEDITATIONS (available August 2008)
FAIRIES 101 (abridged audio book)
GODDESSES & ANGELS (abridged audio book)
ANGEL MEDICINE (available as both 1- and 2-CD sets)
ANGELS AMONG US (with Michael Toms)
MESSAGES FROM YOUR ANGELS (abridged audio book)
PAST-LIFE REGRESSION WITH THE ANGELS
DIVINE PRESCRIPTIONS
THE ROMANCE ANGELS
CONNECTING WITH YOUR ANGELS
MANIFESTING WITH THE ANGELS
KARMA RELEASING
HEALING YOUR APPETITE, HEALING YOUR LIFE
HEALING WITH THE ANGELS
DIVINE GUIDANCE
CHAKRA CLEARING

Oracle Cards (44 or 45 divination cards and guidebook)

HEALING WITH THE ANGELS ORACLE CARDS
HEALING WITH THE FAIRIES ORACLE CARDS
MESSAGES FROM YOUR ANGELS ORACLE CARDS
MAGICAL MERMAIDS AND DOLPHINS ORACLE CARDS
ARCHANGEL ORACLE CARDS
GODDESS GUIDANCE ORACLE CARDS
MAGICAL UNICORNS ORACLE CARDS
DAILY GUIDANCE FROM YOUR ANGELS ORACLE CARDS
SAINTS & ANGELS ORACLE CARDS
ASCENDED MASTERS ORACLE CARDS
MAGICAL MESSAGES FROM THE FAIRIES ORACLE CARDS
ANGEL THERAPY® ORACLE CARDS
ARCHANGEL MICHAEL ORACLE CARDS (Available December 2009)

All of the above are available at your local bookstore, or may be ordered by visiting:

Hay House USA: **www.hayhouse.com®**
Hay House Australia: **www.hayhouse.com.au**
Hay House UK: **www.hayhouse.co.uk**
Hay House South Africa: **www.hayhouse.co.za**
Hay House India: **www.hayhouseco.in**

Doreen's Website: **www.AngelTherapy.com**

To my beloved grandmother,
Ada Montgomery,

who taught me that love comes
not from the stomach,
but from the heart;

that love is not to be feared
or viewed with suspicion,
but is to be welcomed
and nurtured;

and who taught me that the
greatest source of love of
all is from God, who is
ever-present within
each of us now.

BREAK THE PATTERN OF

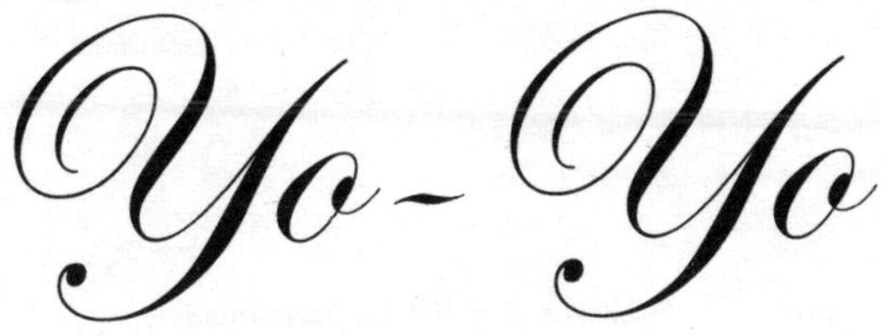

DIETING FOREVER!

How to Heal and Stabilize Your Appetite and Weight

Doreen Virtue PhD

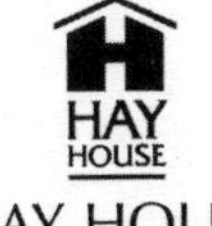

HAY HOUSE
Australia • Canada • Hong Kong • India
South Africa • United Kingdom • United States

First published and distributed in the United Kingdom by:
Hay House UK Ltd, 292B Kensal Rd, London W10 5BE. Tel.: (44) 20 8962 1230;
Fax: (44) 20 8962 1239. www.hayhouse.co.uk

Published and distributed in the United States of America by:
Hay House, Inc., PO Box 5100, Carlsbad, CA 92018-5100. Tel.: (1) 760 431 7695 or (800)
654 5126; Fax: (1) 760 431 6948 or (800) 650 5115. www.hayhouse.com

Published and distributed in Australia by:
Hay House Australia Ltd, 18/36 Ralph St, Alexandria NSW 2015. Tel.: (61) 2 9669 4299;
Fax: (61) 2 9669 4144. www.hayhouse.com.au

Published and distributed in the Republic of South Africa by:
Hay House SA (Pty), Ltd, PO Box 990, Witkoppen 2068. Tel./Fax: (27) 11 467 8904.
www.hayhouse.co.za

Published and distributed in India by:
Hay House Publishers India, Muskaan Complex, Plot No.3, B-2, Vasant Kunj, New Delhi –
110 070. Tel.: (91) 11 4176 1620; Fax: (91) 11 4176 1630. www.hayhouse.co.in

Distributed in Canada by:
Raincoast, 9050 Shaughnessy St, Vancouver, BC V6P 6E5. Tel.: (1) 604 323 7100;
Fax: (1) 604 323 2600

A catalogue record for this book is available from the British Library.

Revised and updated edition; previously published in 1997, ISBN 978-1-56170-352-4

ISBN 978-1-4019-1572-8

Printed and bound in the UK by CPI William Clowes Ltd, Beccles, NR34 7TL.

"One must eat to live,
not live to eat."

— Jean Moliere (1622–1673),
French playwright

CONTENTS

APPENDICES

PREFACE

When I wrote the first edition of *Break the Pattern of Yo-Yo Dieting Forever* in 1988 (originally called *The Yo-Yo Syndrome Diet)*, I felt as if I were stepping out on a window ledge poised high above a busy intersection. I was risking my psychotherapy career and reputation by saying that emotions and stress—not fat and calories—were the true culprits behind obesity. My stance was based upon many years of personal and clinical experience with overeating.

As I was writing the book, my eating-disorder clinic was filled with clients who had dropped many pounds through the use of psychotherapy, and there was a waiting list of people hoping to enter the clinic. Yet, for all that success, the original edition of this book was initially met with scepticism when I went out on a book tour to promote it. Nonetheless, the book became a best-seller and was published in four languages. It was also one of the first psychology books about weight control ever published in Japan.

That was twenty years ago. Today, it is well known that overeating is a mechanism of the mind and emotions. New research on brain chemicals such as serotonin and cortisol, and their links to appetite, promises exciting new answers to the mind–body link in weight control.

In my Hay House books about compulsive overeating: *Losing Your Pounds of Pain: Breaking the Link Between Abuse, Stress, and Overeating;* and *Constant Craving: What Your Food Cravings Mean and How to Overcome Them*, I introduced another area related to appetite: the spirit. My spiritual background stems from being raised by a mother who was a Christian Science practitioner, and by my witnessing miraculous physical and emotional healings through the use of prayer.

Over the years, I have blended the spiritual healing methods that I learned at my mother's knee with the psychological training I received from my university training and clinical practice. This book blends scientific research, my clinical practice results, and the beautiful healing help of *A Course in Miracles*. The *Course* uses the term "God" with male pronouns. If this bothers you, please feel free to substitute a gender-neutral pronoun in your mind, or use the term "Creator" or other synonym for God.

The result is a very effective balance of body–mind–soul therapy that helps my clients attain confidence and inner peace. When you are at peace, your appetite naturally stays low and stable. Your weight naturally drops, because you are not overeating. This method, like most things in life that work well, is very simple.

Doreen Virtue, PhD

ACKNOWLEDGEMENTS

This is the fourth book that I have written with the Hay House team, and my affection and admiration for my publishing family grows with each new book. It is an honour and a joy to work with Hay House.

This book and my work would not be possible without the loving instruction and influence of my mother, Joan L. Hannan; my grandmother, Ada Montgomery; and my great-grandmother, Pearl Crane. Thank you to my father, Bill Hannan, for always encouraging me to write.

I am very grateful for the research help provided by Robyn Ridley, BN, of Crystal Clear Reflections in Australia. Robyn was instrumental in ensuring that the latest scientific research supports this book's premises.

I also want to acknowledge those readers of my books who have written to me and attended my workshops over the years. Your heartfelt correspondence and enthusiastic seminar participation are my greatest rewards for writing these books. Thank you!

PART ONE

THE HUNGRY HEART

CHAPTER ONE
THE YO-YO DIET SYNDROME

"A normally-minded person will eat normally. If one is a glutton, it is because his mentality is filled with unexpressed longings, which he is trying to sublimate."

— Ernest Holmes (1887–1960),
author of *The Science of Mind*

Gina, a 42-year-old brunette, tried all the diets, and none of them worked for her. "I need to lose 30 pounds, but I just keep putting more weight on!" she told me. Gina was desperate to lose weight. Standing 5′6″ tall, she weighed 175 pounds. She had been on one diet after another since age 15, and she'd lost and gained her excess weight too many times to remember. Gina suffered from the Yo-Yo Diet Syndrome—that is, her weight chronically fluctuated up and down.

For people such as Gina, losing weight has little to do with dieting. She knew, as so many of us do, that weight loss depends upon burning more calories, carbohydrates and fat grammes than are consumed. Like Gina, most of us have read countless diet books and have joined diet clubs; we're *experts* on dieting. Yet, for all this knowledge, we cannot keep the lost weight off! New research shows that people worldwide are more overweight than ever before.[1] Why? Because weight has little to do with the body, and everything to do with the mind and spirit. We use food to relax, as a reward, to procrastinate working on our life purpose, and for short-term relief from fear, stress, or emotional pain.

The Yo-Yo Diet Syndrome is not a physical issue. It is a behavioural response to holding depressing thoughts about oneself and one's life. At one time, a popular notion was that yo-yo dieting caused sluggish metabolisms, and that weight *regains* were natural consequences of continual dieting. New research disputes this theory, however.

A 1994 study released by the National Task Force on the Prevention and Treatment of Obesity published in the *Journal of the American Medical Association* took a group of the country's best and brightest scientists and asked them to review all the research to date about the links between "weight cycling" (the clinical term for the Yo-Yo Diet Syndrome) and health conditions. The scientists concluded that most previous studies about weight cycling had been seriously flawed. For example, some studies compared groups of yo-yoers against "control" groups of people whose weights were supposedly stable. However, we now know that the people in many of the control groups had histories of *extreme* weight fluctuations, which makes any comparison between the groups meaningless!

Previous studies also lacked consistent definitions for "weight fluctuations" or a "yo-yo dieter". The task force concluded:

> *The majority of studies do not support an adverse effect of weight cycling on metabolism. There is no convincing evidence that weight cycling in humans has adverse effects on body composition, energy expenditure, risk factors for cardiovascular disease, or the effectiveness of future efforts at weight loss. The currently available evidence is not sufficiently compelling to override the potential benefits of moderate weight loss in significantly obese patients. Therefore, obese individuals should not allow concerns about hazards of weight cycling to deter them from efforts to control their body weight.*[2]

Because the Yo-Yo Diet Syndrome is rooted in our psychological self-image and not in a defective metabolism, I have always steered my clients away from focusing upon their bodies, weight, or food. Every physical correlation of the Yo-Yo Diet Syndrome can be traced back to psychological roots. For example, studies and my own research show that Yo-Yo Diet Syndrome dieters—especially Binge Eaters—have significantly higher levels of depression and psychopathology than among the general population.[3]

The Yo-Yo Diet Syndrome creates a mad cycle of depression leading to eating, and then eating leading to depression. Compared to the general population:

- ☆ Binge eaters are more likely to see themselves and the world through negative points of view,[4]

AND

- ☆ Binge eaters are more likely to overeat in response to negative emotions.[5]

Fortunately, this negativity can be halted and healed! Instead of seeking to control your appetite and your weight, we'll work on spiritual and psychological ways to take charge of your thoughts so they are more loving, positive and truthful. By changing the framework of your thoughts from fear-based to love-based, negative thoughts and feelings will dissipate, and so will your desire to binge eat.

By pinpointing the issues that kept Gina, the client whom you met at the beginning of this chapter, in her overeating mode, I helped her adopt a healthy relationship with herself, her body, and with food. As a result, her weight dropped naturally, and today there is no reason to believe that Gina will ever be heavy again.

If you are tired of fighting your weight and your appetite, you too can heal your weight. I say "heal" because overeating is a disease-like behaviour that hurts our physical and mental health. Diets are bandages. They mask, but don't stop, the underlying pain that is the root cause of overeating. The only cure for compulsive overeating is to heal its psychological source. Be assured that you *can* heal your weight. You *deserve* freedom from the tyranny of an out-of-control appetite!

What Is the Yo-Yo Diet Syndrome?

The Yo-Yo Diet Syndrome is a pattern of losing and gaining weight over and over again. Women are particularly vulnerable, although men certainly suffer from the syndrome, too. All sorts of attempts are made to lose weight—skipping meals and fasting, exercising and fad diets—but the weight is just a symptom of the true syndrome, which is a sequence of psychological and physical patterns common to Yo-Yo Syndrome dieters.

If you have been on many diets in your lifetime but are currently unhappy with your weight, if you tend to binge on a certain type of food (chocolate, potato crisps, bread, spicy foods, cheese, and so on), and if you eat more when you're angry or stressed, chances are you suffer from the Yo-Yo Diet Syndrome. If so, you know first hand the frustrations of looking for the magical cure that will take your weight off and keep it off for good.

Most diet books and programmes deal with the problem on a purely physical basis, promising that if you combine foods in certain ways or eliminate fats, carbohydrates, refined foods, or dairy products, your excess weight will disappear forever. The limited long-term success of these diet plans is clearly illuminated by the way "new" diets are constantly sought after and are propelled into bestselling books, one after another. If any of these books contained *the* secret to permanent weight loss, there would be no need for new diet books.

These books haven't been permanently adopted by many dieters because they don't address the main reasons that people overeat. In fact, most diets contribute to dieters' food obsessions by asking them to constantly weigh and measure their food, *thus leading to more preoccupation with food and eating than if they weren't on a diet*! These diets are often a lot of work and are difficult to stay on for more than a few weeks or months. What has been needed is a simple, yet effective, way to manage and heal the psychological pain that causes overeating. That method, based upon spiritual healing methods that are successfully used to treat physical and emotional conditions, is detailed in this book.

Some books say it's okay to be overweight. Society is too obsessed with being thin, the authors write, with an underlying message to "stop worrying about your weight so much. You're fine just as you are". While I'm the first to agree that the media have contributed to the national obsession with losing weight, I don't think it's wrong to want to look and feel healthy.

Many scientifically sound studies have pointed out that thin or normal-weight people consistently receive better treatment from strangers, spouses, children, employers and co-workers, compared with the obese.[6] Is this fair? Of course not. But is unfairness any reason to ignore such a strong social bias? In truth, we're probably all prejudiced in favour of aesthetic beauty, whether it means appreciating an attractive body, a breathtaking flower, an impressive mansion, or a skilfully filmed movie.

There's nothing wrong or superficial with wanting to improve your fitness level. Being fit doesn't erase all of life's problems, but in many ways it does make life easier. If you lose the obsession with eating and losing weight, you automatically have more time on your hands. Admittedly, the prospect of having more time frightens some people into diving right back into their bags of crisps. After all, a core reason for overeating is to procrastinate over working on one's life purpose. The Yo-Yo Syndrome dieter tells herself, "I can't start working on my true goals until I lose this weight." The pain involved in procrastinating working on our life purpose, and anguished worries about whether we are *capable* of fulfilling our life purpose, are temporarily quelled by overeating.

If your weight constantly fluctuates, you are paying dearly for it. Your ever-changing fat levels can damage your self-esteem and confidence, your relationships with people, and your pocketbook.

The reasons why people suffer from the Yo-Yo Diet Syndrome vary, so there's no one absolute right way for everyone to heal their appetites. The methods outlined in this book take this individuality into account and offer you ways to match your recovery programme with your unique situation and eating style. Much of what you'll read about in this book will trigger deep feelings. Please don't ignore or cover up these feelings with food! Instead, listen to your heart's guidance, as this is how you will discover your personal pathway to a more healthful and meaningful life.

Break the Pattern of Yo-Yo Dieting Forever combines the therapeutic methods of spiritual healing, psychotherapy and behavioural modification. The goal of *Break the Pattern of Yo-Yo Dieting Forever* is for you to learn simple, effective ways to manage your moods so that your appetite for food stays naturally low. My personal and clinical experiences have taught me one lesson loud and clear: *successful weight maintenance hinges upon maintaining your peace of mind.* Keep your mind and heart at peace, and your appetite stays normal. Your weight naturally follows suit.

All the steps are thoroughly outlined in this book. The steps aren't particularly difficult, but each one is important. For that reason, don't read ahead of yourself. In other words, complete each step as you read it in this book, and read the steps one at a time. Please do the steps in order as you find them, and you will lose weight, be able to keep it off forever, and feel good about yourself spiritually, emotionally and physically.

It's very important that you understand *why* you overeat as a means of finding out *how* to keep the weight off for good. This book is divided into two parts. In the first, you will pinpoint why you overeat and read about spiritual, psychological and behavioural ways to overcome and heal these tendencies. In the second half of the book, you will find many suggestions for lifestyle shifts and changes that go hand-in-hand with permanent weight loss.

A Practical Approach

The information in this book is the product of research derived from several sources. First, my own struggle to overcome the Yo-Yo Diet Syndrome was my difficult initiation into the world of endless diets that never quite lived up to their promises. Somehow, that quick weight-loss answer always seemed to evade me. Second, my work as a metaphysical psychotherapist treating overweight people has enabled me to see firsthand the patterns of Yo-Yo Syndrome dieters. I've spent countless hours with frustrated dieters and have learned what they overeat and why. I've also seen my approach to the Yo-Yo Diet Syndrome work on clients who were convinced that they'd never lose their excess weight.

My work blends eight years of university training in counselling psychology, 13 years of clinical practice, and a lifelong study of metaphysics. I am the daughter of a spiritual healer, raised to use prayer and spiritual principles to heal every seeming problem or difficulty. When I was a little girl, my mother taught me to use affirmations and visualization. Is it any wonder that I lean upon my earliest upbringing in treating the issues of compulsive overeating?

After 13 years of clinical practice, I am convinced that a spiritual approach to eating and weight loss is the most efficient and pleasant choice available. Yo-Yo Syndrome dieters already endure massive amounts of pain. Why inflict additional trauma through the use of conventional dieting approaches, especially when such methods are impotent? The reason why this book emphasizes spirituality isn't to win anyone over to a particular belief system or religious philosophy. Not at all! In fact, many of my clients have suffered from "religion abuse" and hypocrisy, making them fearful and suspicious of religion and spirituality. Yet, because we work together to help them make peace with themselves, their families and their bodies, they have learned how to benefit from the spiritual approach described in this book. Spiritual healing is the *hands-down winner* among all the choices available to the compulsive overeater. It offers a method for completely absolving the inner pain that causes overeating in the first place. If you are tired of struggling with the Yo-Yo Diet Syndrome, I encourage you to give these methods a fair try and see if you agree that they really work.

The information in this book is also drawn from the latest research on obesity. There are some vital facts about brain chemistry that help explain the Yo-Yo Diet Syndrome. The researchers in this field are tracking some very exciting areas that also clarify why most diets aren't effective.

The Yo-Yo Diet Syndrome solutions that I present here have worked for me and for my clients, and they will work for you too, if you study and use the principles.

CHAPTER TWO
SPIRITUAL SOLUTIONS FOR THE YO-YO DIET SYNDROME

"Great men are they who see that the spiritual is stronger than any material force."

— Ralph Waldo Emerson (1803–1882),
American philosopher

Gut feelings are a superb guiding force. They tell us the best routes to take in every aspect of our lives. We've probably all had instances where we regretted ignoring a gut feeling about a job or a relationship. Conversely, you've probably obeyed an illogical intuitive impulse—and were very glad that you did.

Intuition in the form of gut feelings also tells you when to make changes in your life. Your gut may urge you to return to college, read a particular book, change careers, leave a relationship, call a certain person or take up a new hobby. When I was fat and depressed, I felt I wasn't making a contribution to the world. My gut directed me to take psychology classes and to write books and magazine articles about my life's ups and downs. My intuition's directives initially intimidated me, and I would overeat gallons of ice cream to try to silence its ceaseless "change your life, change your life" chants. The ice cream would momentarily ease my existential discomfort. But this satiation never lasted long, and soon

I would face my gut feeling's incessant pressures to make my life healthier and more meaningful.

Finally, I gave up fighting my gut feelings. I enrolled at a local community college and immediately felt relief as my life clicked into focus. My appetite, especially for ice cream, lessened, and my weight started to drop off almost without my noticing. I began writing and submitting articles to magazines. Although they were all rejected, I felt elated that I was following my inner guidance. This energy carried me through 12 years of college and propelled me to keep writing until I eventually had many books and articles successfully published.

I had been afraid to follow my gut feelings. It was easier to not even *try* to work on my inner dreams than face the pain of possible failure, rejection and ridicule. Housework and eating were my escape into a safe world where I couldn't fail. Even though my gut feelings gave me a clear picture of my dream life, I couldn't imagine *how* I could ever attain the life I imagined. Now I know that our gut gives us directives on how to fulfil our dreams just one or two steps at a time. Like a correspondence school, once we complete those steps, we are given the next set of assignments. Our task isn't to look at the end picture. It's to follow our gut feelings' directives on a gradual basis.

Just as I have a life purpose, so do you. You already know, deep down, what your life purpose is. If you are unaware of what it is, it's because fears keep you from acknowledging your intuitive voice. Almost all of my clients initially come to me because their appetite feels out of control. Underneath their voracious appetite is a volcano of fear and anxiety, and most of this stems from an unfulfilled life purpose. As I once did, my clients bury their gut feelings—that rich source of information about their life purpose—under mountains of food, alcohol or addictive relationships. These behaviours are the equivalent of sticking your fingers in your ears and saying to your gut, "I can't hear you! I can't hear you!"

Healing from the Yo-Yo Diet Syndrome involves so much more than the foods you eat or what size clothes you can wear. It involves reconnecting and forming a trusting partnership with your gut feelings.

As you follow your intuitive voice, you will be fully guided to improve many aspects of your life. Some of that guidance may frighten you and require blind faith on your part. Afterward, you'll be rewarded with improved relationships, finances, a sense of meaningful purpose, health, and the sure knowledge that you made a positive difference in the world. The more experiences of this type that you have, the easier it will be for you to unquestionably follow your gut. I will give you specific methods throughout this book to increase your awareness of your gut feelings.

Our intuition is intimately connected with our spiritual self. Spirituality and prayer are becoming more integrated with traditional methods of healing physical disease and illness. Today, many physicians pray for their patients' health, and hundreds of well-documented medical studies show that prayer significantly helps the healing process.[1] It is no different with the condition of overweight and overeating. Prayer heals the anxiety and depression that lead to eating binges.

The Ego's Appetite for Pain

Your true self doesn't overeat or think obsessively about food. Your true self isn't concerned with your weight or appearance. And your true self doesn't feel guilty or anxious about food. However, the part of you that overeats feels hungry all the time, worries, feels guilty and insecure, and that broods about diets and pounds is your *ego*. Actually, the ego isn't even part of you because your true self—also known as your higher self—is the only being created by God (or spirit), and therefore the only being who is real and eternal.

The ego is the part of us that *appears* to be real because we give it so much attention. However, since the ego is not a part of God, it is inherently unreal and temporal. Once we release the ego, the desire to overeat naturally subsides. I want to spend some time discussing the mechanics of the ego mind, because it's necessary for you to recognize when you've slipped into your ego.

What it boils down to is that, any time you feel any pain, you are in your ego state of mind. Your true self knows only complete peace and love and is oblivious to pain because it is unreal. It is *very* important, in order to recover from the Yo-Yo Diet Syndrome, to take the time to really understand the difference between the true self and the ego. Here is a chart that shows the main differences:

EGO	TRUE SELF
Pain	Love and bliss
Unreal, temporal, destructible	Real, eternal, indestructible
Worries, fears, doubts	Is patient, nonjudgmental, good-humoured
Guilt and fear of punishment	Innocence, peace, calmness, gratitude
Uses judgment	Uses intuition
Miscreates and schemes	Has unlimited creativity, ideas, enthusiasm
Competitive, believes in limited supply	Win–win, cooperative, a giving spirit
Holds grudges	Forgives
Fears the inner voice	Welcomes and follows the inner voice

Our attention is like a laser beam. It can only be on one side or the other, in the ego or the higher self. It cannot be on both sides simultaneously. Symptoms of being in the ego include feeling less than or greater than another person, or feeling scared, guilty or insecure.

Another example is if you feel frustrated because you work so hard in meditation to attain inner peace, only to feel pulled off your spiritual path when you get out into the "real world". This occurs because a resentment or judgment has pulled you back into your ego.

The ego was created when you and I decided, in a moment so long ago that it is buried in our subconscious, that we would prefer to be separated beings. Like teenagers wanting their own apartments, we wanted separation from God and from one another. We decided, at the moment of separation, that we didn't trust the Creator to make our decisions for us. We desired our own universe apart from the Creator where we were in total control. Some of us did this out of fear of an "angry God", and some of us did this out of arrogance, desires for experimentation, or rebellion.

Our higher self knows that the ego is insane and that it is impossible and totally undesirable to separate from God. Why would we want to leave our source of joy and love? However, the ego is invested in keeping us miserable, because as long as we forget how perfect and beautiful we and all our brothers and sisters are, the ego can rule the roost. The ego knows that if we remember Divine Love, we will no longer pay attention to the ego's ravings.

The ego tries to con us into believing that if we feel guilty enough, we'll be vindicated for all the pain that has been inflicted upon us by all the "horrible people". Such thoughts keep the separation real and solid in our minds. Also, if you feel guilty, you expect punishment to be inflicted. You then *create* situations of attack in your life—perhaps by orchestrating a crisis at work or home, or attacking yourself with self-deprecating thoughts. (This in no way implies that a person who abuses you is not responsible for his or her behaviour.) The bottom line is that all forms of attack stem from the ego's guilt out-pictured into the world.

What does this have to do with overeating, and recovering from the Yo-Yo Diet Syndrome? *Everything*! First, many studies and my own clinical research show that negative thoughts and emotions are a major instigator of eating binges. A person comes home from work and mentally replays the day's events. Maybe she decides she didn't work hard enough that day or that her co-workers don't like her. She says to herself, "No one understands me; I'm no good at anything I do," or some other put-down of herself. These words put the key in the ignition of the ego. Pretty soon, she feels tired (ego conflicts result in fatigue) or inferior to others (a prime characteristic of the ego).

At the same time, her true self's inner voice tries to dissuade her from these self-recriminations by saying something like, "Go to the art store and buy some painting supplies. Your true purpose is in the artistic endeavours that you always loved to do in the past. You will be helping many people with your creations." This inner voice scares her. She feels intimidated—"How could I possibly have anything to contribute to the world, let alone as an artist? I have no talent!"

She shuts off the inner voice's promptings and instead responds to the ego's call to punish herself for her "guilt". The ego seductively promises that if she punishes herself enough, she will be liberated from pain and futility. This is the ego's lie that so many of us have fallen prey to. But we don't have to, because the ego's bark is huge, and it has no bite unless we buy into its false promises.

Looking on the Outside

When we listen to our ego's voice, we take our focus off our inner wisdom. Other people's opinions matter more than our own. Our concerns about what people might think keep us from trying new ventures. We eat when the clock tells us it's lunchtime, even if we don't feel hungry. The ego turns us away from our intuition, which creates a personality style known as "extroversion".

A majority of compulsive overeaters fall into the personality category of "extroverts". Extroverts can be wonderful socializers who are warm and thoughtful. It is not "bad" or "good" to be an extrovert; it is simply a style of relating to the world.

The difficulty that extroverts have with food is that they get hungry because of external cues—the sight of food or because the clock says it's noon, for example—instead of relying on internal cues that it is time to eat, such as hunger pangs. One study even found that extroverts' insulin levels rise at the mere sight of food, which in turn increases their hunger. Other research has discovered that extroverts are more likely to eat high-fat and highly sweetened foods, and that they report experiencing more pleasure while eating, compared with introverts.[3]

From a spiritual standpoint, I find that extroverts often attempt to fulfil desires for love through externals such as shopping, eating, dating, or even reading. None of these activities is harmful; however, they only give *temporary* happiness. This is in contrast to the consistent levels of contentment found through daily prayer, meditation, and communion with your Higher Power.

Diets are another external source leading to temporary happiness. Whenever a new diet book comes out, many people fall into a hypnotic spell of believing, "This is it! This is the answer I've been seeking!"—that is, until they become bored with the diet plan and abandon it for the next weight-loss craze.

Spiritual solutions to the Yo-Yo Diet Syndrome require filling one's emptiness with something that lasts. It means committing to a spiritual path that helps you lose the fears and anxieties that make you want to overeat. We each must find and follow our own spiritual path, and it's important to trust your intuition to lead you to teachings that ring true and that—most important—are devoid of fear.

Taming the Desires of the Flesh

Every major spiritual and religious school teaches that material desires are the downfall of those seeking inner peace and lasting happiness. Many spiritual works emphasize that we can avoid bodily temptations by keeping our focus on spirituality. For example, the Apostle Paul wrote, "Walk in the Spirit, and you shall not fulfil the lust of the flesh."

We often face temptations that distract us from our highest priorities—desires that seem like shortcuts to bliss. Yearnings for sex, money, fame, prestige, appeals of vanity, and gluttony pull us away from our true purpose. These material objects aren't inherently wrong, bad or evil. It's just that when we obsessively desire them, we are pulled away from the spirit. Material objects never give us the rewards we were certain would lie there. Instead, earthbound trappings coax us in a very addictive way.

That's why we struggle with our desire to eat! Food diverts our attention from difficult tasks or pressing worries. Food is a less threatening alternative to working on our major goals. We know we won't fail or be rejected while we're eating. We're not so self-assured about the unknown landscape of a new career, relationship or venture. So we choose food as a safe haven of comfort, a place where we know nothing is difficult or trying.

After overindulging in food, we may feel guilty or anxious. Part of this is concern over the calories consumed. But overeating leads to emotional hangovers because we know, deep down, that we could have applied the time spent eating to much better use. We feel so much better investing even 15 minutes toward our major goal, instead of on some fleeting pleasure such as eating.

When I procrastinate, my intuition nags at me like a bill collector; however, it leaves me alone as long as I'm involved in some meaningful activity such as meditation, nature walks, playing with my kids or my cat Romeo, reading or writing. But let me prolong plucking my eyebrows, watching mindless television or staying on the Internet too long, and my intuition badgers me with a palpable roar.

In the old days, I would silence my intuition by grabbing whatever food was handy. Sometimes, I'd drink wine on top of the food to put an extra seal on my inner voice. I hated being told what to do, even when I knew the advice was coming from my higher self and was in my own best interests. Overeating was my rebellion against the loving guide who was coaxing me to work on my true purpose.

Somewhere along the way I lost the ability to lie to myself. Now, I can no longer get away with ignoring my inner guidance. None of the old methods—overeating, shopping, socializing, primping or preening—have the power to completely block my awareness of my purpose.

Am I now miserable that I no longer languish in the sanctuary of overeating? Not at all. My true sanctuary is where yours is: within my choice to hold only peaceful thoughts and retain a loving outlook. That is how I now get full.

The Purpose of Your Yo-Yo Diet Syndrome

All situations are potential lessons that help us grow and prosper. In a sense, your Yo-Yo Diet Syndrome is a gift because it has compelled you to increase the awareness of your intuition and your life purpose. By letting go of overeating, you naturally hear your gut feelings. By following those gut feelings, you automatically feel better about yourself and your life. Fulfilling your life purpose puts your entire life in sync. Fortunately, the more time you put into your life purpose, the more your appetite normalizes. Your weight and the food you consume cease being the darlings of your awareness, and the pounds drop off.

How Overeating Blocks Your Purpose

We each have a purpose in life. It is the unique contribution we make to the world with our natural talents, interests and passions. We can fulfil this purpose with our career, volunteer work or a special project. The form our purpose takes isn't so important. However, it *is* important to identify and work on our purpose without delay.

Our purpose gives meaning and a benevolent structure to our lives. Some people have vague ideas about their life purpose, but fears and insecurities keep them from taking action. Those who haven't identified their life purpose feel lost, as if they are forgetting to do something important—which they are.

We are driven to make a difference in the world. This drive is powerful and pervasive—as much a force of nature as the wind that carves canyon walls and the surf that pounds shorelines. Finding and living our true purpose is a simple and natural process. Like the proverbial bird in the hand, we already have everything we need in order to fulfil that purpose.

However, our ego may convince us that our natural talents and abilities couldn't possibly be valuable enough to make a difference to the world. We wrap those judgments around our true self like an eggshell, to shield it from hurt and rejection. Our purpose then sits trapped and unfulfilled while we search outwardly for what we already have.

We can't completely ignore the awareness of our unfulfilled purpose because our true self's voice, the intuition, hounds us with reminders as if we have an unpaid debt. We may muffle the volume of this intuitive voice through extreme behaviours such as overeating or alcohol abuse. We may procrastinate working on our purpose by stuffing our schedules with meaningless activities. We may pretend that we don't care that our talents and true interests lie dormant and unused.

However, no ego-based fears or behaviours can completely silence the inner voice, and delaying our purpose creates depression and anxiety. Our only route to inner peace and fulfilment is to hear and follow the intuitive guidance that drives us to discover and work on our life purpose.

We don't need to add anything to ourselves to tap into our intuitive voice or to release our inborn purposeful talents. We only need to *subtract* the ego's fears and distorted viewpoints from our consciousness. Once we do so, we readily hear and follow the intuition's guidance as to the nature and direction of our purpose. Fortunately, all we need to do to release the bird in our hand is to make a tiny crack in the ego. Nature then takes over in the rebirth of our true self and all of its gifts.

People who fulfil their purpose through their careers wake up excited about their work and say, "It's wonderful that I'm being paid to do something I love!" Their material and financial rewards—which are usually plentiful due to their spirited dedication to work—are icing on the cake.

Yet, many people feel unable to have a purposeful, enjoyable career. They know the theories about "following your bliss". However, their ego binds them with paralyzing guilt, insecurity and fear. They feel undeserving of happiness and don't believe it's possible to have a fun job, or they feel guilty that they're making money with their talents. These pervasive ego-based feelings bar them from even dreaming about, let alone starting to work toward, improving their life and career. That's why silencing the ego voice and amplifying the true self's intuitive voice is *essential* to fulfilling your purpose, transforming your work life and enjoying the freedom of authenticity.

I was involved with clients who have healed their lives for 13 years in private practice and in two inpatient psychiatric programmes I directed. I firmly believe that unfulfilled life purposes are the cause of many psychological maladies. My clinical theory is that people use extreme behaviours such as overeating and alcohol abuse as "delay tactics" for procrastinating their purpose. They use substances as a way of ignoring their intuitions' urges to make changes in their careers or home lives. Although these changes would improve the quality of their lives, they initially resist their inner guidance. They feel undeserving of happiness or unqualified to turn their true interests into a career. They are afraid to trust and follow their intuition, so they try to muffle the volume of their gut feelings by pouring food on their gut. They also overeat to cover awareness of the pain and emptiness that come from ignoring their purpose.

I help my clients identify and trust their intuition because I believe that we are all inherently intuitive, and anyone can learn how to increase their intuitive powers. I teach my clients how to access their intuition's instructions about fulfilling their life purpose. Just by taking small steps, the client's desire for overeating or other extreme behaviours dissipates, and any depression or anxiety is relieved.

The ego is our only block to identifying and fulfilling our purpose. It is the element that blinds us to knowing our true self as unlimited, ingenious and loving. If we could always hold the knowledge of our true perfection steady in our consciousness, our intuition would naturally guide us to our purpose. However, the ego pulls us down and makes us feel inadequate, afraid, guilty and undeserving of happiness. It's unrealistic to expect to escape the ego's clutches completely, because everyday events at work and at home trigger our fears and insecurities. What we *can* do, however, is learn how to identify and escape from our egos quickly.

Once we learn how to stay centred in our true self, we naturally become more aware of and more trusting of the gut feelings that lead us to and along the path of our purpose. If we stay out of the ego, our purpose is naturally apparent! Without the ego's grip, we readily hear and obey the intuitive voice, and our purpose unfolds almost effortlessly.

Many of my clients initially resist creating an enjoyable life built around their natural interests. They don't believe they deserve, or can make sufficient money with, a pleasant life and a meaningful career. I help them heal ego beliefs such as, "Life should be a struggle," or "I don't deserve happiness."

I also call certain types of ego traps "delay tactics". These are the meaningless activities and nonexistent problems that we create to procrastinate fulfilling our true function. We tell ourselves, "I'll get started on what I'm *really* supposed to be doing with my life right after I'm done with this project, or after I lose ten more pounds."

Yo-Yo Syndrome dieters procrastinate by using their weight or eating as a hedge against the perceived "danger" of facing the task of fulfilling a purpose. We can identify and heal delay tactics through complete self-honesty, listening to our intuition, committing to our purpose, and by asking for spiritual intervention.

Shedding the ego involves nothing more than recognizing when you're in this state of mind. It's like noticing you've taken the wrong exit off the highway of your life purpose and true self-state. Berating yourself for the mistake isn't helpful. Instead, you must get back on the road.

To live in our true self-state fully, we've got to be free of ego judgements. The true self is our natural state, and we needn't add anything to ourselves to get there. We must, instead, subtract all ego beliefs that tell us that we are separate from others and from our Creator. The act of forgiveness is central to shedding the ego because resentment and thoughts of retaliation feed the belief in separation. Forgiveness increases the volume and clarity of the intuitive voice.

Forgiveness also boosts self-confidence and a belief in oneself.

Adopt a "Zero Tolerance for Pain" Policy

On a table near my meditation area, I have a sign that says "PAIN". Around the word is a circle that is diagonally slashed with a thick line. The sign is my reminder that I have a "Zero Tolerance for Pain" policy. I teach my clients this policy, and I urge you to adopt it for yourself.

Like the "Zero Tolerance for Drugs" policies in many public schools, my no-pain policy is a way of committing myself to never allowing any emotional pain refuge within my soul or body. Pain is not an idea or creation of God's; it is purely human-made. I don't want any loveless thoughts in my mind, and neither do you, believe me! Yet, it is very easy to overlook one or two painful thoughts. Then before you know it, your mood feels like you're at the end of a very long and dark tunnel and you can't find your way out to the light. It's so much easier to train yourself to notice when you feel the slightest bit of emotional pain. Evict it immediately, or it will invite its other no-good friends to reside within you!

Does this mean ignoring or denying the pain? No, because that would just substitute spirituality for food in stuffing down the pain. Besides, each of the painful "problems" in our lives contains valuable healing lessons. They teach us awareness and hopefully convince us to let go of our blind spots, prejudices, tendencies to ignore our intuition, and other growth lessons. You don't want to miss extracting this information from your pain by pretending it doesn't exist.

Instead of advocating stuffing down pain, I'm recommending turning it over to Heaven. This involves bravely facing the pain and the problems head-on and saying to them, "I will not accept you in my life. Go away now, but leave your valuable insights behind on your way out."

Any time you're feeling pain to any degree—from a minor irritation all the way to a desire to kill—you are in your ego state. You feel pained, afraid and alone because you have momentarily lost your awareness of the connection between yourself, all other beings, and with your Creator. If you were raised to believe in an "angry God", you may also be afraid of retaliation.

If you feel emotional pain, it's not wise or helpful to deny its existence. The key is to non-judgementally acknowledge the pain, such as, "I notice that I'm afraid right now" or "I feel betrayed." Don't judge your pain as bad or good—such labels solidify and enlarge the pain. And you don't want that to happen!

The spiritual text *A Course in Miracles* offers the most effective solution to emotional pain that I've ever found. This method gives nearly instantaneous relief and healing to any type of pain, trouble or problems. It truly is a one-size-fits-all solution, since there is no order of difficulty in miracles. Our ego tries to convince us that some problems are larger than others. However, problems actually have no mass or size. During my years of study and clinical practice, I've had the opportunity to study and try just about every psychological method, including the medical model, behaviourism, humanistic, Jungian, Gestalt, cognitive, and logotherapy. Many of these methods work, some of them don't, and most of the traditional solutions provide temporary relief at best. Most of them are very time-consuming.

Here's the *Course in Miracles* prescription that I teach my clients and use for myself:

Know that emotional pain is a product of your ego. Since your ego isn't real (in the sense that God didn't make it and it is destructible), its effects are also unreal. There are two ways to undo this pain. The long way is through analysis and introspection. A shorter, more efficient way is like asking a professional housekeeper to come into your house and clean up a mess. The housekeeper here is the Holy Spirit. If for whatever reason the name "Holy Spirit" bothers you, please substitute a name you feel comfortable with such as "Spirit", "Love", "The Voice of God", "The Universe", or "The Force". Some of my clients prefer "The Holy Housekeeper".

This ever-present power of God knows exactly how to return our house to orderly peace by rapidly correcting our thoughts until they align with perfect truth and love. Without a trace of judgement about the mess our ego made, the Holy Spirit comes in like a whirlwind, cleans us up, wishes us blessings, and leaves us completely restored.

The first step is to quiet your mind and silently ask the Holy Spirit to return you to a peaceful state. The second step is to be receptive to the help. If you called a housekeeper but refused to let her enter your home, she'd be quite ineffectual. If you told her, "Don't look at the mess that I made," how could she clean it up?

So it's important not only to ask for Holy Spirit's help in correcting your thoughts, but also to open the door so Holy Spirit can enter and do the work. Don't hang on to even one scrap of useless ego product—give it all to the Holy Housekeeper. Be sure to thank Holy Spirit afterward for the miraculous cleaning job.

Here is the method, based on *A Course in Miracles*, that I teach all my clients (who come from every religious and non-religious background) to instantly relieve any ego pain or seeming problems:

First, take a deep breath and close your eyes. Imagine holding your pain or problem in the hand that you write with (this is your releasing hand), and say,

> *"I am feeling emotional pain. I know this pain isn't true, since it is not from Love, and Love is all that is true. So I must have chosen a wrong thought. I want to feel peace instead of*

pain. Please enter my mind now, and help me to see this situation in another way. Please correct all my thoughts so they are in alignment with Divine truth. I ask that all effects of mistaken thinking be forgotten in time by everyone involved."

In less than a minute, you'll feel a shiver or shudder in your body. Some people call this Kundalini energy, and the *Bible* refers to it as "the wind"— don't worry, it's perfectly safe. I think of it as the Holy Spirit giving my soul a chiropractic adjustment to bring my thoughts into alignment.

Next, expect a miracle. The power of this method is so all encompassing that it triggers changes in the outward appearance of all situations. Remember that everything mirrors our thoughts through the Law of Cause and Effect. Change your thoughts, and your world also changes.

When a new client is honestly and completely willing to release their weight and eating to Spirit, their appetite is often healed in one session.

"The monster that was inside me always demanding to be fed is no longer there. It's a miracle!"

"I've lost ten pounds in a month without even thinking about it. My friends tell me I look ten years younger!"

"I almost don't want to tell you this, because I'm afraid of jinxing it, but after one session, I no longer get up in the middle of the night and binge."

These are among the actual testimonials I have received from clients who were willing to be spiritually healed from overeating. Their appetites normalized after just one session because they were ready to be healed. If you can let go of all fears of giving up control of your eating and your weight to God and the angels for *just one instant*, Spirit will receive your invitation to enter and heal your mind and heart. Heal the hurt, and you heal your weight.

When we stop trying to control situations, we open the channel for Divine, perfect will to heal our lives. Invariably, our sights are set much lower than Heaven's, so surrendering to God's will always results in better-than-expected outcomes. All parts of the so-called problem will transform in loving and miraculous ways. As it says in *A Course in Miracles*:

> *You whose mind is darkened by doubt and guilt, remember this: God gave the Holy Spirit to you, and gave Him the mission to remove all doubt and every trace of guilt that His dear Son has laid upon Himself. It is impossible that this mission fail...The Holy Spirit offers you release from every problem that you think you have. One mistake is not more difficult for Him to bring to truth than is another.*

In this world of free will, we must ask for help. Without our express invitation, the Divine won't intervene, except in a dire emergency. Remembering to ask for help is often the most difficult part of spiritual healing! After you request help, God takes care of everything else.

PART TWO

THE FIVE OVEREATING STYLES

CHAPTER THREE

RECOGNIZE YOUR YO-YO DIET SYNDROME STYLE

"A well-governed appetite is a great part of liberty."

— Lucius Seneca (4 B.C.–A.D.65)
Roman philosopher

There are five overeating styles in the Yo-Yo Diet Syndrome. Each has a different emotional, metaphysical and behavioural cause. You may recognize yourself in more than one (or in all five) of these overeating styles. Take a moment now to single out which kind of Yo-Yo Syndrome dieter you are: "The Binge Eater", "The Emotion Eater", "The Self-Esteem Eater", "The Stress Eater", or "The Snowball Effect Eater".

1. *Those Who Can't Stop Eating Certain Foods*—**"The Binge Eaters".** Becky, who prided herself on always being organized and "together", couldn't understand why she lost control and went on a binge every time she ate something with chocolate in it. Similarly, JoAnn found that she couldn't keep a quart of ice cream in her freezer without finishing it off in one sitting. Chocolate, sweets, bread, salty junk foods, ice cream and frozen yogurt, nuts, cheese, creamy salad dressings, and spicy Italian or Mexican dishes are very common binge foods.

2. *Those Who Use Food for Comfort*—**"The Emotion Eaters".** Janice's high-pressure job put her in many upsetting situations, yet she had difficulty telling people that she was irked by their behaviour. After work, Janice would have a whole day's worth of anger stored up inside her, and as soon as she got home each evening, she would head right for the refrigerator to feel better.

   In addition to being used as a cover-up for anger, food is used to combat feelings such as fatigue. Cindy felt exhausted after a day of chasing her toddler and caring for her newborn baby. To give herself enough energy to prepare dinner each evening, she'd eat sugary snacks such as candy or cookies and wash them down with a cola.

3. *Those Who Use Food to Feel Better About Themselves*—**"The Self-Esteem Eaters".** Hillary put her husband and kids first and spent what little extra money the family had on *them*—never on herself. She wore old knit pants and ragged shirts, and she often forgot to put on make-up. In the ten years of her marriage, Hillary gained over 80 pounds because overeating was another way that Hillary mistreated herself.

4. *Those Who Use Food When They're Under Stress*—**"The Stress Eaters".** Rosalyn, a middle-management executive at an insurance company, never felt as if she had enough time to get everything done. "I put in 50 hours a week at work," she says, "then I have to come home and take care of my family. My weekends are spent doing laundry and grocery shopping—my only 'fun' seems to be when I eat!"

   Unfortunately, Rosalyn's choice to use food as a stress-management tool had resulted in a 30-pound weight gain over the past 2 years. "Before I took this job, I had a lot of pride in how I looked," Rosalyn explained. "But now, I just don't have any time to exercise or go to a diet club! I've almost resigned myself to the fact that I'm going to end up being fat like my mother was."

5. *Those Who Gradually Increase Their Food Consumption*— **"The Snowball Effect Eaters".** Diane had been gaining and losing the same 15 pounds as long as she could remember. "It never fails," she explained. "I'll no sooner get the weight off than I'll start putting it back on again!" On closer examination, we found that Diane would lose weight by cutting the size of her meals. Once the 15 pounds were off, Diane would stop paying attention to her portions, and her meals would grow larger and larger until she put back on all the weight.

   Every winter, Darlene, another Snowball Effect Eater, would put on 20 extra pounds. "At least I can hide it under bulky sweaters and coats," she told me, "but it sure would be nice to stay the same weight year-round for once in my life." Each spring would find Darlene vigorously dieting and exercising to prepare for summertime and bathing-suit season, a pattern she was extremely tired of.

Every style of Yo-Yo Syndrome dieter stems from an attempt to mask the pain of not fulfilling one's life purpose. However, each style has a particular form of fear that blocks the purpose's manifestation. In the following five chapters, I have listed the metaphysical meaning for each Yo-Yo Diet Syndrome style. I have also prescribed an affirmation for each, as one antidote to the fear that creates the desire to overeat. I recommend that you write the affirmation for your style (or styles, if more than one applies to you) on a 3-by-5 index card, and post it in a place where you will be certain to read it two or more times every day. Within 30 to 40 days, this affirmation will loosen many of the hardened fears connected to your overeating style. If you combine the affirmation with the suggestions in Chapter Two and the recommendations given in the chapter corresponding to your eating style, you have all the tools necessary to permanently heal your appetite and weight.

If you find that you suffer from a combination of Yo-Yo Diet Syndrome styles, then it's a good idea to pay attention to the Yo-Yo Diet Syndrome steps given for all the styles that apply to you. In fact, most Yo-Yoers are able to see themselves in all five of these styles from time to time. For that reason, I'd recommend reading all the material in this book as you begin your programme.

No matter what type of Yo-Yoer you are, please know that you *can* finally achieve your ideal weight—and maintain it—without yo-yoing.

CHAPTER FOUR
THE BINGE EATERS

"It is impossible to seek for pleasure through the body and not find pain...It is but the inevitable result of equating yourself with the body, which is the invitation to pain."

—A Course in Miracles

Each of the five eating styles of the Yo-Yo Diet Syndrome has specific characteristics. Here are the particular eating tendencies that apply to style number one: The Binge Eater.

☆ The Binge Eater tends to overeat one or two particular "binge foods"—such as bread, chocolate, cheese or salty snacks.

☆ Once the Binge Eater has one bite of their binge food, their eating habits and appetite go out of control.

☆ The Binge Eater sometimes worries, often without justification, that she won't get enough to eat.

☆ The Binge Eater goes to extreme lengths (for example, driving several miles out of her way; spending excessive money, and so on) to obtain the binge food.

The metaphysical basis of binge eating is a belief in lack, and a fear that there isn't enough good (or food) to go around. The Binge Eater fears that by the time she discovers and fulfils her life purpose, someone else will have "beaten her to it" and she won't be needed in the world.

The affirmation for the Binge Eater is:

> *"There is an unlimited supply of good for me and for everyone else. My life purpose is uniquely mine, and it is important that I make this contribution without delay because life's orchestra depends upon the harmonious blending of all individuals."*

The Binge Eater really doesn't want to overeat; she feels *driven* to do it. Pamela, for example, wanted to refrain from eating sweets more than anything. But invariably when she'd go into the kitchen, she'd think about the cookies in her cupboard.

> Pamela struggled to stay away from the cookies, thinking, *No, I won't eat them!* Then she'd think, *Well, just one won't hurt*, so she'd head toward the cupboard—and then stop herself with a *No!* Then she'd say to herself, "Yes, I do deserve to have one." The more she fought with herself, the more anxious she'd become. The more anxious she became, the more she wanted a cookie. After a few more minutes of this war being waged within her, Pamela knew that eating a cookie would calm her down. She grabbed the cookie bag before she had time to talk herself out of it. Chewing away, Pamela sighed with relief.

Pamela's eating was compulsive, because she really didn't want to eat the cookies. It's one thing to willingly choose to eat a cookie, but quite different to struggle with yourself and then feel defeated after giving in to the overpowering urge to eat.

> Another client of mine, Audrey, experienced a different sort of pain connected to her Binge Eater style. When Audrey's husband complained about her binge eating, she laughed. "I thought he was jealous of the way I could eat anything I wanted," she remembered, "but I hadn't let myself notice that I'd put on 35 pounds in 2 years." Audrey denied her problem with food because she held on to a major misconception about overeating. "I thought Binge Eaters were those people who ate everything in sight for three hours and then threw it all up," she said. "I wasn't doing that, so I thought I wasn't bingeing."

Whenever you eat for reasons other than physical or emotional hunger, you are technically binge eating. You don't have to eat a refrigerator full of food to be on an eating binge. A binge can consist of eating just one cracker if that cracker is compulsively eaten. If you don't really want to eat that cracker but feel compelled to eat it anyway, then your eating is out of control.

> Melanie, a dark-haired, well-groomed 27-year-old secretary, was able to control her eating during breakfast and lunch. But when she got home at four o'clock, she'd head straight for the refrigerator and compulsively search for something sweet to eat.
>
> "I'd pull out a carton of ice cream and promise myself I'd eat just one spoonful," Melanie explained. "But that first one would taste so good that I always ended up having another. And then another. Sometimes I'd eat half the carton before realizing what I'd done."
>
> Melanie's four o'clock binges eventually put 30 extra pounds on her, and she knew that she'd have to cut out the sweets in order to successfully lose weight. She was incredibly frustrated by the time she came into my clinic for help

> with her Yo-Yo Diet Syndrome. "I just can't get by until dinner without overdoing my eating!" she complained.

Melanie was out of control over ice cream—it was her binge food. A binge food is any substance that makes you want to eat more and more. Every Binge Eater's binge food is different, but it usually consists of sweets such as chocolate, cookies, candy, ice cream or frozen yogurt; salty junk foods such as nuts or potato chips; spicy foods such as Mexican, Italian or Thai dishes; cheeses and sauces; or bread products. Here are two other examples of clients who were Binge Eaters:

> Rhonda was a late-night Binge Eater whose binge food was potato crisps. Every night she'd unwind in front of the television set with a bag of crisps and some salsa or dip. Although Rhonda would try to eat just three or four crisps, she'd always finish the bag and go on to eat pretzels, crackers or popcorn. Every morning Rhonda would promise herself that she'd stay away from the salty junk foods... only to break the promise that evening.

> A 38-year-old homemaker, Candace always put off eating her first meal until the kids were off to school. Then at 10 o'clock it was time for her favourite game show, and she would fix buttered English muffins to eat during the hour to come. All too soon, her favourite show would end, and Candace would be left with a two-storey house to clean. To put off that mundane task, she'd toast more muffins—crunchy-brown, with pools of butter. They comforted her when the rest of the day's activities seemed drab or depressing.

For Melanie, Rhonda and Candace, overeating was triggered when they ate their binge foods. Melanie's ice cream, Rhonda's salty junk foods and Candace's muffins had the same effect: they made these women feel better, and that feeling led to desiring more. Yo-Yo Diet Syndrome Binge Eaters are unable to stop eating once they taste their binge food. Even after months of dieting, and after all the work that went into losing weight, one taste of a binge food destroys their efforts, and their weight yo-yos one more time.

If you are a Yo-Yo Diet Syndrome Binge Eater, you may have identified your particular binge food, but to help you really get a clear picture of the scope of this phenomenon, the next section will explore the nature of common binge foods.

Step #1 for Binge Eaters: Identify Your Binge Foods

Some Binge Eaters have no trouble identifying their binge food. They know without a doubt that they can't eat just one cashew or one brownie. Other people say that *all foods* are their binge foods, and it certainly can seem that way when you overeat at every meal, every day. I've found, though, that Binge Eaters have at least one particular food that triggers an eating binge. If you're a Binge Eater, the first step in healing your Yo-Yo Diet Syndrome is to identify what your binge food is, for reasons that are discussed later in this chapter. The descriptions below may help you to identify that food.

While reading them, ask yourself these questions:

- ☆ How does eating this food make me feel? Calm or energized, happy or sad? What other emotions does it trigger in me?

- ☆ Have I ever been able to eat just one piece or bite of this food? Do I want more the next day or later that week?

- ☆ When I eat this food, do I feel guilty or nervous afterward?
- ☆ How many times have I begun an eating binge after taking a bite of this food?

Chocolate

"Chocoholic" has found its way into the English language with a tongue-in-cheek connotation attached. For many Binge Eaters, though, chocolate is no laughing matter due to the way it keeps weight constantly fluctuating. Let's say you decide to diet in time for the holidays. After three or four months of rigorous self-discipline and losing twenty or thirty pounds, you feel really good about the weight loss. Then the holidays come—and with them, the inevitable boxes of chocolate candy.

Feeling foolish over worrying about "just one piece of chocolate", you reach for the candy box and find you cannot stop with just one piece. You say, "Well, I've blown my diet for this day, so I may as well indulge." At that point, an eating binge ensues. It may begin with chocolate and end up with any other type of food that happens to be in the vicinity.

Recent studies help to explain why some of us crave chocolate. First, chocolate contains powerful stimulants that lead to a sudden surge of energy right after it's eaten. Second, chocolate contains a chemical called *phenylethylamine* (P.E.A.), which is identical in molecular structure to the P.E.A. produced by the brain during states of "romantic love". I've noticed that my clients who are having marital or dating difficulties have stronger cravings for chocolate than they had before the relationship problems. Their desire for chocolate is actually a craving for feelings of love. This observation was recently backed up by a study showing that "chocoholics" have higher-than-normal tendencies to fall in love easily and be devastated by romantic rejection.

In addition, hormonal fluctuations make many women crave chocolate before and during their menstrual cycles.

Finally, if the other chemicals weren't enough, the *aroma* of chocolate contains another mood-influencing substance called *pyrazine*. When inhaled, pyrazine activates the pleasure centre of the brain, leading to feelings of contentment. Many chocoholics try to control their cravings by switching to low-fat chocolate treats. However, it's easy to rack up a 1,000-plus calorie binge by consuming a box of low-fat fudge brownies. Better methods to reduce chocolate cravings are discussed in Chapter Nine.

Other Sweets

Some Binge Eaters aren't tempted by chocolate at all, but are drawn toward other sugary desserts. Candy, cookies, doughnuts, ice cream, pies, cakes and even soda pop are all difficult for dieters to resist, but if this is your binge-food category, staying away from these desserts can seem almost impossible. For example, my client Sylvia was a dessert binger who really had a weakness for doughnuts. Every morning, she'd stop by the doughnut shop under the guise of picking up a two-dozen box for her coworkers, but she would always eat half the box or more.

Sylvia had to face the reality that she was actually buying the doughnuts for herself, not for the people at work. Sugar gives the body a large boost of adrenaline and leads to feelings of euphoria and high energy. The high soon topples, however, leading to a slump in emotion and energy levels. Then, the cravings for more sugar begin.

Sweet desserts are also loaded with another substance connected with mood-regulation: carbohydrates. Carbohydrates activate a brain chemical called *serotonin,* which produces a calming effect and reduces feelings of depression. It appears that some people are more sensitive to carbohydrate-induced serotonin than others.

One study showed that the same amount of carbohydrates can make some people feel jittery and anxious, while making others feel calm. Sugary desserts such as pies, cookies and cake often contain more carbohydrates than some chocolate foods, which may explain why some people can leave chocolate alone but can't stay away from other sweets. How you react to carbohydrates depends on your chemical make-up, and since everyone's brain chemical levels are different at various times of the day as well as everyone's mood preferences—some people prefer to be calm, while others like to be more energetic—it makes sense that everyone's binge foods are different.

As with the other common binge foods, this is merely an explanation of why you may prefer sugary foods. Some realistic solutions for your cravings are described a little further on in this book.

Salty Junk Foods

Nuts, pretzels and potato crisps appeal to Binge Eaters who crave foods that are crunchy and high in fat. People who overeat when they're angry or stressed tend to pick crunchy foods on which to take out their aggressions. Christina, for example, was continually upset at her husband for not pitching in around the house. She'd come home from work and find him asleep on the couch while the children ran around the house unsupervised. Usually she'd console herself by munching on a bowl of buttered popcorn or some potato crisps. As she voraciously crunched away, her anger toward her husband would usually subside.

In addition, studies now show that overeaters have a "fat tooth" as well as the proverbial sweet tooth. In other words, many overeaters crave fat in the foods that they choose. One reason is that fat stays in the stomach longer than other foods, leading to a sense of fullness for a greater length of time. Salty junk foods have an extremely high fat content, and people whose binge food is in this category have a hard time cutting back because their stomachs are accustomed to holding a certain amount of fat. Yo-Yo Syndrome dieters who attempt to stay away from salty junk foods may feel hungry all the time and thus be tempted to eat "just one" crisp, nut or pretzel. But as with the other binge foods, there's no such thing as "just one". The first three days are the most difficult when cutting back on fat, so hang in there, because it soon gets easier.

Those who binge on nuts are also attracted to the chemical pyrazine in their aroma. The vapours of pyrazine trigger the pleasure centre of the brain, leading to feelings of enjoyment as you smell or eat the nuts. People who are fun-deprived often binge on nuts as a means of chemically compensating for their all-work-and-no-play lifestyles. This, of course, adds to the binge-food properties of this food because it's tough to break away from something that makes you feel good. And since chocolate contains pyrazine, chocolate-covered nuts are a particularly common binge food.

There is also a physiological need to chew a certain number of times every day. If this need isn't satisfied—for instance, if you eat only soft or creamy foods—it can lead to cravings for something crunchy to gratify that urge to chew. You can fulfil that need by chewing carrots, celery, frozen fruit pops or whole-wheat crackers.

Dairy Products

While you may turn to crunchy foods because you're angry, cravings for soft dairy products such as cream cheese, ice cream, frozen yogurt, dressings and sour cream often signal a desire for comfort when you feel sad. Sandy, a 32-year-old homemaker and mother of three, continually craved buttermilk "ranch-style" salad dressing. She poured the dressing on practically everything she ate, and she'd even eat the dressing by the spoonful.

Dairy products do have a satisfying texture to some Yo-Yo Syndrome dieters, and they also contain a number of chemicals that reduce depression and lead to feelings of calmness. For instance, dairy products have high amounts of L-tryptophan. This amino acid is a precursor (catalyst) for serotonin, the brain's mood-regulating chemical. But in order for L-tryptophan to fully metabolize in the brain and bring on the strongest relaxation effect, carbohydrates must be present with the dairy product. This chemical combination may explain why many people binge when they eat cheese with crackers, bread, pizza or tortillas, as well as other dairy product/carbohydrate mixtures.

Dairy products also contain large quantities of *choline*, a substance that spurs production of a brain chemical responsible for feelings of happiness and contentment. This binge-food category, as with the others, is full of mood-altering chemicals.

Breads and Starches

One thing I noticed in my years as a psychotherapist is that many people are in occupations involving their binge food. My client Harold, for instance, couldn't have been in a worse job for someone whose binge food was bread: he drove a bakery truck! Imagine that, if you will. Harold's binge food constantly followed him around for nine hours at a time. Not surprisingly, he finally decided that controlling his weight meant leaving the bakery business.

People turn to bread, pasta, rice or potatoes because the high carbohydrate content of these foods increases the brain's serotonin levels. This leads to calm, happy feelings. In addition, the yeast and glucose in breads are both stimulants that provide mood and energy boosts. The boost, however, is soon followed by a drop in blood sugar, causing low energy levels and mild depression. The vicious cycle of overeating bread and other starches begins when Binge Eaters eat more of these foods to feel good again.

Bread is a difficult binge food to contend with, because it's such an intrinsic part of mealtime. Not only is bread served as a side dish at most restaurants, but every kind of meat imaginable is breaded. Pasta, closely related to bread, is also combined in many salads and main dishes. Most bread bingers are able to curtail their cravings by eating other forms of starch at their meals, such as rice, corn or potatoes.

Spicy Meals

Spicy meals such as Mexican, Italian, Cajun or Thai also consist of common binge foods.

> Helena, for example, always knew that Mexican food was the downfall of her diets. Every time she'd lose weight, she'd have to avoid burritos, tacos and tostadas—not due to the calories or fat grammes in these foods, but because she couldn't stop eating them once she started.
>
> She'd go to a taco stand and promise herself, "I'll just have one." Then, as she stood at the order window, she'd smell the aroma of spicy beef and melting cheese and end up ordering two or three burritos. "I'd be so embarrassed about ordering that much food for myself that I'd order two sodas so the restaurant employees wouldn't think it was all for me," Helena remembered.

Mexican and Italian meals that combine aged cheese such as Parmesan or cheddar, with yeast-laden tortillas, pizza crusts, noodles, and beef or chicken, are loaded with the chemical tyramine. This powerful stimulant leads to mood and physical energy elevations almost immediately after the food containing it is eaten. The boost is readily followed by a low, of course, and the overeater begins craving more food to feel good again.

People who overeat spicy foods often have high thresholds for excitement and crave a lot of stimulation in their lives, relationships and meals. Those attracted to spicy foods also tend to take emotional or physical risks, create crises, and generally "live life on the edge" because they crave such a high level of drama.

Extremely hot-flavoured foods such as chilli peppers are craved by people feeling overwhelming emotional pain. In many cases, they have recently suffered a huge loss, usually the death of a parent. Their unresolved grief is so painful that they eat chillies to trigger the brain's production of cortisol—a natural pain anaesthetic chemical. (I discuss the links between emotional pain and overeating in my book *Losing Your Pounds of Pain.*) I will talk about how to resolve and manage grief and unhappiness in later chapters of this book.

Of course, the compulsion to overeat spicy foods is also triggered if your binge food—say, cheese or bread—is an ingredient in the meal. In such cases, spicy foods may not be your actual binge food. You can tell by looking at your preferences. Do you enjoy a mild flavour of your favourite food, but in a pinch you will eat a spicier version if that's the only thing available? Or do you have a "the-spicier-the-better" philosophy? Do you tend to salt your foods before you taste them? If you answered yes to the first question, then you're not likely a spicy food binger. A yes answer to either of the last two questions, on the other hand, means that you are a spicy food binger.

One way that spicy food Binge Eaters can control bingeing behaviour is by increasing the sensitivity of their taste buds. To do this, stay away from alcohol, caffeine and cigarettes for at least one hour before eating. Drinking water, especially with a lemon or lime slice, will help keep your palate cleansed and reduce your desire for highly spiced meals.

Health Foods

For some, health foods are a binge-food category. Although this may be surprising to you, health foods contain many of the same mood-elevating chemicals as other foods. No food is either good or bad—the important question is whether or not the food triggers a binge in *you*.

> My client Peggy was a highly educated woman who prided herself on her knowledge of health and nutrition. She collected books on the subject and did most of her shopping at farmers' markets and health-food stores. Her diet consisted of natural food, uncontaminated by pesticides, salt or refined sugar.
>
> But Peggy still suffered from the Yo-Yo Diet Syndrome because she binged on health foods. "They taste so good and make me feel so good, too," Peggy complained. "I just can't stop eating them!" She'd binge on dried fruit, carob drops and granola bars.
>
> Upon examination of Peggy's eating habits, we found that her binges occurred when she ate foods sweetened with highly concentrated natural forms of sugar. The fructose in dried fruits and the honey in granola bars triggered binges in Peggy.

Health-food bingers such as Peggy are usually bingeing on natural forms of some of the common binge foods named above. Whether it's refined or natural sugar, chocolate or carob, fat-free or fat-filled, if a food makes you binge, then it's your binge food. Health-food bingers need to find patterns in the particular type of food they're overeating. If it's in the dried fruits or natural-candy category, then the section on "Other Sweets" on page 39 may offer some clues. If it's granola, then look at the "Breads and Starches" section on page 42. If the binges occur in response to raw nuts, read the section on "Salty Junk Foods" on page 40.

Identifying Your Binge Foods

Your unique personality, chemical make-up, experiences with the food, and personal taste preferences will decide which foods you turn to most often. My book *Constant Craving* goes into even greater detail about the reasons we crave certain foods. Which foods are your binge foods? For some people, it may be two or three of those mentioned above.

If you're not sure what your binge food is, consider the following:

- ☆ Do you consistently crave a certain type of food?
- ☆ When you eat it, do you have overwhelming urges to eat more?
- ☆ Is it difficult for you to stay away from that particular food?
- ☆ Do you find yourself craving more of the food a day or two after you eat it?
- ☆ Do you want to eat this food even when you're *not* upset and there's no stress in your life?

If you answered yes to at least three of these questions, then the food in question is your binge food. If you answered yes to only one or two of the questions, the food may not be a binge food but may still place you at high risk for a binge. Some people are not able to pinpoint what their binge foods are right away because they've never really paid attention to their reactions to particular foods. If you're still unsure what your binge food is, then take one or two weeks to carefully study your own eating behaviour. The best way to do this is to keep a written log of what you eat and your feelings before and after you eat each food. Admittedly, this requires a lot of work, but it will focus your attention on your reactions to different foods.

If you don't care to keep a food journal, then try to make your meals distraction-free (for instance, don't watch television, read, or drive while eating), and eat each different food on your plate one at a time so you'll be able to distinguish how each food makes you feel. Pay close attention to your anxiety levels as you eat each food. How do you feel when you eat the dressing on your salad? Do you want more and feel as if you can't get enough of it? How about your dinner roll or pasta? How do you feel when you're eating dessert?

Look for patterns in your eating, and you'll see what your binge foods are. Of course, others who regularly eat with you may already have a good idea what foods you binge on, so you might want to ask them their opinion on this subject.

Intuition Integration for Binge Eaters

Your inner voice and your spiritual support will help you prevent or overcome overwhelming urges to eat, and also help keep your appetite in check. There is always a moment of conscious choice right before making the decision to binge. During that moment when you think, "One little taste of my binge food won't hurt," or "I've already eaten my binge food so I may as well keep eating," remember to think of and listen to your intuitive voice. Even an instant of hearing the loving reasoning coming from your intuition can be enough to return your mind to sanity.

In addition to the suggestions given in Chapter Two about calling upon spiritual strength and support, it's also a good idea to "go within" frequently throughout the day. Please don't wait until your cravings or your eating have gone out of control, although spiritual intervention does work even in the midst of an all-out binge. However, you are kinder to yourself when you remember to ask for help the moment that you feel your desire to gorge kick in.

Remember to keep a "Zero Tolerance for Pain" policy. The moment you start mentally tasting your binge food, or the second you feel yourself losing control of your appetite, go within—you can even do this when a part of you really wants to keep eating and doesn't want your appetite to be healed. Have the sane part of your mind ask this question: "What is my hunger trying to tell me?" Your intuition is probably urging you to notice something, or to take some action. Deep down, you already know what your intuition is trying to say. But fear has made you turn from acknowledging its wise counsel.

Many Binge Eaters avoid listening to their intuition because they fear that they will have to exert some energy, when inside they feel burned out. I have found that many Binge Eaters are paralyzed with beliefs that this is a competitive world and that "I better get mine before someone else gets it first." This is often rooted in childhood experiences of having to compete for food at the dinner table. However, Binge Eaters believe that this lack of good extends to all life areas. They are concerned that there is not enough love, money, appreciation or health to go around. By confronting the illogical nature of this deep-seated belief system, Binge Eaters can learn to relax about their food supply. This is an important step in healing desires to binge eat.

Most important, however, is that letting go of uptight fears about lack enables the Binge Eater's intuitive voice to be heard. Fear obliterates its volume and prevents Binge Eaters from hearing and benefiting from its guidance. I have found that Binge Eaters, who are unaware of their intuition during conscious waking hours, do very well to consult their dreams for sources of inner guidance. I highly recommend that all Binge Eaters keep a blank journal and pen next to their beds to capture this rich supply of information. Everyone dreams—even those who swear they don't.

You will remember your dreams by writing this sentence on a piece of paper and putting it under your pillow: "I ask to have a dream that I will easily remember and that will clearly give me guidance about how I can attain more happiness and peace of mind." Mentally repeat this sentence before falling asleep. In the morning, before doing anything else, write down whatever memory fragments of dreams you have. As you write, you will remember more and more. Write whatever you get, and then ask your higher self to explain the dream's meaning and relevance to your life.

Your dreams and intuition will guide you through every aspect of your life if you let them. You can easily distinguish between your intuitive voice and the voice of the ego because the former is a calm and loving voice of reason, while the latter involves phrases that are put-downs and insults. For instance, the intuition would say, "I know I can write a book that will truly help people. I feel guided to enrol in a writing course at the adult school to help me get started."

The same message coming from the ego would sound like this: "Everybody wants to write a book! Who am I to think I'm qualified to write? What could I possibly say that would be original enough? By the time I get around to writing a book, someone else who is more qualified will have already written about my topic, but with a better writing style."

If you made decisions based on the ego voice, you would act out of fear and tension. Our inner voice that urges us to fulfil our purpose doesn't go away just because we ignore it or cover it up with food. Only by following the intuitive voice that encourages you to write a book, take photographs, become a healer, or whatever is part of your purpose, can you be assured of attaining the peace of mind and meaningfulness you are truly craving.

Breaking Away from Binge Foods

If you are able to control your eating when you're calm, and only binge on food when you're upset, then you are not Binge Eating—you are Emotion Eating (which is described in Chapter Five). Binge foods, in contrast, remain triggers for binges *even when you're feeling calm, relaxed, and at peace with yourself.* This is because the binge food's mood- and energy-altering chemicals are creating an allergic-type reaction that triggers anxiety. A paired-association response has been created—first in the mind, and then transferred into the body's cellular memory. Once the Binge Eater tastes the binge food, the body's autonomic nervous system becomes aroused in a fight-or-flight response. The ensuing anxiety from eating the binge food then leads to out-of-control eating.

Fortunately, there is a way to break this paired association so that the binge food can be enjoyed in moderation. Binge Eaters are well-advised to completely abstain from their binge foods until the conditioned response is broken. As Saint Augustine said, "Complete abstinence is easier than perfect moderation." Instead of struggling with trying to control the eating of your binge food, why not avoid it entirely until you have worked through the underlying issues that trigger your binges?

So, to repeat: eating binges need to be avoided at all costs. They put the weight back on us after months of working at getting the pounds off. They make us feel bad about ourselves, because after a binge we feel guilty, weak and out of control. One of the best ways to avoid bingeing—until your appetite and weight are healed—is to avoid those foods that are clearly your binge foods.

On the other hand, if you're able to eat just one piece of a certain food, or if you overeat only when you're experiencing a "fattening feeling" (see Chapter Five), then you need not eliminate that food from your diet. In other words, if you can eat one piece of candy, one biscuit, one potato crisp or one cookie, and you do not feel compelled to voraciously consume the rest, then you can eat that food and still lose weight. Similarly, if you only binge on these foods when you're upset, then you'll have to avoid them only during the times when you're feeling emotional and vulnerable to overeating.

If you're a Binge Eater, as you progress through the steps of breaking the Yo-Yo Diet Syndrome, you will be able to add your former binge food back into your meals if you choose. For now, your task involves paying close attention to your reactions to the foods you eat. Notice what foods you binge on, and look for any connections that your hunger pangs and cravings seem to have with emotions or stressors in your life.

By paying attention to both the mind and the body, the steps involved in healing the Yo-Yo Diet Syndrome provide the tools you need to achieve permanent weight loss. In Chapter Five, we'll look at style number two in the Yo-Yo Diet Syndrome: The Emotion Eaters.

CHAPTER FIVE
THE EMOTION EATERS

"They whose sole bliss is eating can give but that one brutish reason why they live."

— Juvenal (A.D. 60–140), Roman satirist

Emotion Eaters are often at a loss to explain why the pounds they've lost creep back again, and they may blame themselves for their lack of willpower. But, in truth, it's really a lack of self-awareness that's to blame—not being aware of what it is that drives them to eat so much. Here are the characteristics of style number two in the Yo-Yo Diet Syndrome:

☆ The Emotion Eater only overeats when she's feeling a strong emotion, such as anger or depression.

☆ The Emotion Eater frequently overeats immediately after getting home from work.

☆ The Emotion Eater tends to eat whenever she is bored.

☆ Sometimes, out of the blue, the Emotion Eater finds that she is incredibly hungry, and she almost feels as if she's starving for food.

☆ The Emotion Eater usually feels uncomfortable openly displaying or talking about her feelings.

The metaphysical basis of emotion eating is a belief that other people keep interfering with her attempts to fulfil her life purpose. She believes that if only her children, neighbours, boss, co-workers, teachers, parents and lover would cooperate, she could get to work on her purpose.

The affirmation for the Emotion Eater is:

> *"I am the sole creator of my life. I choose now to put loving, creative and consistent energy and enthusiastic effort into discovering and fulfilling my life purpose. I take total responsibility for structuring my time."*

One of the main "problems" that Emotion Eaters face is that they feel hungry a great deal of the time. Their solution in the past has been to eat every time they felt hungry. Unfortunately, since they were so often hungry, this meant that they would eat a lot of food and gain a lot of weight in the process.

Step #1 for Emotion Eaters: Identify Your Fattening Feelings

If you are someone who eats to quell emotions, it's important, at this point, to start paying attention to your feelings of hunger. What you'll probably discover in doing so is that much of what you've labelled hunger is actually something else—anger, boredom, fatigue, depression or loneliness.

There are huge differences between emotional hunger and physical hunger, as the chart that follows outlines:

The Eight Traits of Emotional Hunger

Emotional Hunger	*Physical Hunger*
1. *Is sudden.* One minute you're not even thinking about food, the next minute you're starving. Your hunger goes from 0–60 within a short period of time.	*Is gradual.* Your stomach rumbles. One hour later, it growls. Physical hunger gives you steadily progressive clues that it's time to eat.
2. *Is for a specific food.* Your cravings are for one certain type of food, such as chocolate, pasta or a cheeseburger. With emotional eating, you feel that you *need* to eat that particular food. No substitute will do!	*Is open to different foods.* With physical hunger, you may have food preferences, but they are flexible. You are open to alternative choices.
3. *Is "above the neck".* An emotionally based craving begins in the mouth and the mind. Your mouth wants to taste the pizza, chocolate or doughnut. Your mind whirls with thoughts about your desired food.	*Is based in the stomach.* Physical hunger is recognizable by stomach sensations. You feel gnawing, rumbling, emptiness, and even pain in your stomach with physical hunger.
4. *Is urgent.* Emotional hunger urges you to eat NOW! There is a desire to instantly ease emotional pain with food.	*Is patient.* Physical hunger would prefer that you ate soon, but doesn't command you to eat right at that very instant.
5. *Is paired with an upsetting emotion.* Your boss yelled at you. Your child is in trouble at school. Your spouse is in a bad mood. Emotional hunger occurs in conjunction with an upsetting situation.	*Happens out of physical need.* Physical hunger occurs because it has been four or five hours since your last meal. You may experience light-headedness or low energy if overly hungry.

6. *Involves automatic or absent-minded eating.* Emotional eating can feel as if someone else's hand is scooping up the ice cream and putting it into your mouth ("automatic eating"). You may not notice that you've just eaten a whole bag of cookies ("absent-minded eating").	*Involves deliberate choices and awareness of the eating.* With physical hunger, you're aware of the food on your fork, in your mouth, and in your stomach. You consciously choose whether to eat half of your sandwich or the whole thing.
7. *Does not stop eating in response to fullness.* Emotional overeating stems from a desire to cover up painful feelings. The person stuffs herself to deaden her troubling emotions, and she will eat second and third helpings even though her stomach may hurt from being overly full.	*Stops when full.* Physical hunger stems from a desire to fuel and nourish the body. As soon as that intention is fulfilled, the person stops eating.
8. *Feels guilty about eating.* The paradox of emotional overeating is that the person eats to feel better, and then ends up berating herself for eating cookies, cakes or cheeseburgers. She promises to atone ("I'll exercise, diet, skip meals, etc., tomorrow").	*Realizes eating is necessary.* When the intent behind eating is based in physical hunger, there's no guilt or shame. The person realizes that eating, like breathing oxygen, is a necessary behaviour.

(Chart from *Constant Craving: What Your Food Cravings Mean and How to Overcome Them*, by Doreen Virtue, PhD, published by Hay House, Inc., 1995)

Emotion Eaters must become acutely aware of their motivations for wanting to eat. You need this awareness in order to tell whether your stomach's actually empty or you're upset about something and just want to eat to feel better. First, spend the next week analyzing the feelings you have when you're hungry. The best way to do this is to keep a journal recording how you feel before, during and after eating. The journal is a black-and-white way of finding patterns in the emotional reasons why you overeat.

Second, the next time you feel like eating, ask yourself if you could possibly be upset instead of hungry. Don't go to the kitchen automatically when you feel hunger pangs. Instead—and this is important—give yourself a mandatory 15-minute "time out" whenever you think you're hungry. (In Part Three of this book, you'll learn wonderful ways to heal the underlying emotions that make you want to eat.)

Listed on the following pages are the 16 feelings that Emotion Eaters most often confuse with physical hunger. Be as honest as you can with yourself when reading this list, because self-awareness is a key ingredient in recovering from the Yo-Yo Diet Syndrome. These listings merely describe the fattening feelings and explain why they lead to overeating.

1. Anger

Anger is cited in more cases of overeating than any other emotion. Anger, especially when it's repressed, feels very uncomfortable, and this discomfort is often confused with hunger. But what feels like hunger is actually a desire to use food to *cover up* or *mask* the painful emotion—anger.

Women, in particular, have difficulty admitting that they are angry, due to societal pressures ranging from parental admonitions ("Young ladies shouldn't get angry!") to corporate game-playing rules ("You'll get ahead in this company if you just smile and agree with management instead of arguing about their policies."). With all this pressure, people sometimes wish they never felt angry—a futile wish, of course, since everyone gets angry at times. People run into trouble with their anger when they ignore their angry feelings or pretend they don't exist, hoping the emotions will subside if they're ignored long enough. Emotion Eaters turn to food in order to stuff their anger.

Barbara was an Emotion Eater who overate in response to repressed anger. For the first month of dealing with her Yo-Yo Diet Syndrome, Barbara would come into her counselling sessions with me and cry about her overeating and excess weight. It was always apparent from Barbara's tightened fists, her tense, shrill voice and her quick, self-conscious movements that the 37-year-old hair stylist was quite angry—and this is why she overate.

After listening to her talk, I'd say something to Barbara such as, "How were you feeling right before you ate the cake?" "Oh, I don't know," she'd answer. "Okay, I guess... well, maybe just a little upset, too."

"Were you angry at all?"

"No! Of course not! Why would I be angry?"

"Well," I'd reply, "just suppose you were angry. What would you be angry about?"

Barbara eventually admitted to herself that she was angry. Most of her anger centred around what she perceived as someone's thoughtlessness—some instance in which Barbara felt victimized but unable to defend herself. She'd be very angry at the "perpetrator"—usually her husband, boss or mother, but felt she couldn't express or resolve her anger. Her frustration would cause her to eat cake and doughnuts to block awareness of her uncomfortable emotions.

Barbara learned how to heal the source of her anger, using the methods you'll read in this book. After several months of practising these self-healing techniques, Barbara was no longer eating in response to anger.

2. Fatigue

If anger is the number-one psychological reason why people overeat, fatigue is definitely number two. That's why I call it "fat-igue". Some late-night overeaters use food in a vain attempt to energize themselves when they're tired. Shift workers, those who stay up late at night and "workaholics" are especially prone to overeating when fatigued.

Other people use food to calm the nervous tension associated with fatigue. Perhaps you've had a nerve-wracking day at the office, combined with overconsumption of caffeine or chocolate. At night, you try to sleep but find you're too wired. That's when cravings for carbohydrate snacks occur, because these foods trigger calming brain chemicals that help you sleep.

When we're tired, our resolve to eat lighter and healthier foods often goes out the window. Feeling fatigued, we say, "To heck with calorie counting!" and down a quart of ice cream or a massive plate of spaghetti.

It's important to recognize fatigue in yourself when it occurs. Learn to recognize how it feels when you're emotionally drained or intellectually overstimulated. Once you can label these feelings as fatigue, you won't be as likely to confuse them with hunger.

Second, remember that when you're tired, rest will make you feel better. Overeating will not. Food may give you a temporary surge in blood sugar that is reminiscent of feeling rested, but the key word is that the respite is *temporary.* What's more, an eating binge can lead to sluggish, tired feelings the next day as your body tries to break down the high levels of sugar, fat and carbohydrates from the binge foods. Rest, regular exercise and the mind–body methods described in later chapters are the best ways to combat feelings of fatigue. Food only makes things worse!

3. Depression

When life looks gray and gloomy, most Emotion Eaters start to think of ways to feel better, and their solution to depression usually involves food. People who eat when they're depressed often turn to dairy products such as ice cream (particularly chocolate) and cheese. As precisely as a well-trained pharmacist, but intuitively, the overeater picks food that alleviates depression. After all, the chemical make-up of dairy products has a neurological effect similar to antidepressant medications.

> Thoughts about cheese melted on pizza or tortillas crept into Katie's mind almost every day as she struggled to keep up with her children and still manage to complete her housework. Between the cheddar on her daily omelette and the melted Monterey jack or mozzarella on her lunch and dinner menus, Katie would consume nearly a pound of cheese per day.
>
> It didn't take long to discover that Katie's fattening feeling was depression. She felt discouraged and defeated, it turned out, because she had dropped out of college after her marriage, giving up her dream of an acting career.
>
> Married to a trucking-business owner who regularly worked 12-hour days, Katie saw her role in life as being little more than an unpaid housekeeper. She was angry at her husband and resented her kids, but at the same time felt guilt for harbouring these feelings. So, she held them inside and turned the anger inward, at herself. The result was depression and a big appetite for cheese.

Once Katie stopped allowing herself to be a victim—no one was forcing her to relinquish her acting dreams, after all—she returned to acting classes and resumed work on her goals. By restructuring her life to suit her heart's desires, Katie was able to lose 25 pounds and look forward to her future!

Depression occurs for a number of reasons. It can be traced to:

- ☆ Holding in anger (as Katie did).
- ☆ A loss, such as losing a job, getting a divorce, selling a house, becoming ill, or losing loved ones (including pets).
- ☆ Physical exhaustion or poor nutrition. This type of depression readily responds to rest and a healthful diet.
- ☆ "Kicking yourself" and focusing on real or imagined negative characteristics in yourself. Try to keep your attention focused on your positive qualities, and remember that everyone makes mistakes. Forgive yourself!
- ☆ Feeling like a helpless victim and seeing the future as hopeless. You're not a victim, and the future will be as pleasant or as painful as you set out to make it! You really do create your own life.

4. Loneliness

Even though Donald worked in a huge hospital employing hundreds of workers, he felt very alone. Assuming he could trust no one, Donald rarely revealed anything of a personal nature to his fellow employees. An Emotion Eater, Donald turned to food when he felt lonely: baked goods; nuts such

> as cashews, peanuts and sunflower seeds; and peanut-butter sandwiches. These high-fat bulky foods seemed to fill the void in Donald's life—for a few moments. The pyrazine in the nuts triggered brain chemicals that are associated with having fun, which Donald was truly craving. But the more he'd eat and the more weight he'd gain, the more alienated from others he'd feel.
>
> When Donald entered therapy, he was convinced that others didn't like him because he was overweight. Donald couldn't have been more wrong. He had to face the fact that it was Donald who didn't like himself, and that he pushed others away from him. Food and fat were just symptoms to cover up his underlying feelings of being unloved and lonely. Once Donald learned to love and accept himself and began to trust other people, his appetite for peanut-butter sandwiches decreased.

Those who eat out of loneliness usually must push themselves to meet new people, even when the prospect seems frightening. Some of the easiest ways to get out and become active with others involve engaging in some sort of organized group activity, such as joining a volleyball team or a mastermind group, enrolling in any sort of class, or becoming a member of a charitable organization.

5. Insecurity/inadequacy

When I started working in the counselling field, I felt inadequate a great deal of the time. I worked in a large inpatient alcoholism hospital, and we were terribly understaffed. There was always a crisis of some sort with a patient or staff member, and there wasn't much that any of us counsellors could do to keep the atmosphere positive. There was a pervasive air of gloom and despair hanging over us. And always, at the end of the day, I was left with the feeling that I just hadn't done enough to help the alcoholics and drug addicts in our facility. I'd feel empty and at a loss, and I'd want to eat as a result.

Long-term experience as a counsellor and my spiritual background eventually helped me to change my perspective. As you may know, feeling "not good enough" is an empty sensation. The insecurity and inadequacy that come with self-doubt can feel like a big, black empty hole right in the middle of your gut. It feels uneasy. It doesn't feel good. I think that these feelings are among the toughest to contend with because most of us don't even want to admit we're experiencing them. I know that, at times, I used to believe that I was the only person in the world who felt inadequate. And I used to be afraid that merely admitting these feelings—even to myself—might make it true that I *was* inadequate. So I hid the feelings from myself and others and tried to fill the empty hole with food.

Inadequacy is a very normal feeling! *Everyone*, including PhDs, MDs, rich folks and other successful and famous people, wrestles with self-doubt and feels like a failure at times. Problems arise when Emotion Eaters try to ignore or cover up the sense of inadequacy with food, instead of taking steps (such as returning to college, asking for a raise, praying, etc.) to minimise the basis for the feeling.

6. Guilt

> Kim, a divorced mother of two, was unemployed and worried about meeting next month's expenses. She also felt that she'd let her family down because the children needed new school clothes, and Kim couldn't afford any. Kim's gnawing conscience and guilt led her to overeat macaroni and cheese and other pasta dishes.

Another client of mine, Tisha, felt guilty because of her extramarital affair. When she first became involved with her lover, Tisha didn't think that sneaking around to hotel rooms would bother her. But four months into the affair, Tisha began to eat chocolate non-stop as her guilt over the infidelity mounted.

Eating, of course, doesn't resolve a guilt-producing situation. Both Kim and Tisha had to take action at the root of their problems in order to alleviate their guilt. For Kim, this meant cutting down on expenses such as long-distance calls and clothes so she'd have enough money to provide for her children until she could find work. Tisha started to feel more relieved when she broke up with her lover and brought her husband in for marriage counselling.

Besides taking steps to solve the problem, the realization that you are not completely responsible for others and that you truly can't control anyone else's actions or feelings can also free you of unnecessary guilt. This doesn't mean that you have to be thoughtless, just that you can let go of the erroneous notion that you're responsible for the happiness of those around you. No one person is that powerful! Give others credit for the direction they choose to take in their lives.

7. Jealousy

Julia was jealous that her ex-boyfriend, Bob, was dating another woman. She imagined the couple dining and dancing in elegant restaurants, and she tortured herself with fantasies of Bob buying his new girlfriend extravagant and romantic gifts. Although he had been quite unromantic and unimaginative when Julia was dating him, she was sure that Bob would be the perfect lover with his new girlfriend.

> Julia was certain that this other woman was prettier, thinner, smarter and sexier than she herself could ever hope to be. This obsessive jealousy led Julia to nervously snack on cream-filled chocolate cookies, one after another. She'd pace and eat, eat and pace.
>
> To break this cycle, Julia's Yo-Yo Diet Syndrome solution included having her face the fact that Bob was now dating another woman. Julia also came to terms with the realization that Bob was probably just as unromantic with his new girlfriend as he had been with her. And, most importantly, she learned to stop putting herself down and comparing herself to others.

Many "jealousy eaters" I've treated tend to compare themselves unfavourably to others in a process I call "comparing your insides with other people's outsides". This happens whenever you look at other people who *appear* to be so together, happy and confident, and compare this with how you *feel* on the inside. You may become jealous if you assume someone else's life is much better than your own because on the outside he or she appears happier than you do. Remember that outside appearances can be deceiving, and that to other people, you too probably appear to have it all together.

8. Happiness

> Kelly was a "happy overeater". After a year of financial problems and family illnesses, she was relieved when things finally started to go her way. Within two months, Kelly got a raise, her mother's cancer went into remission, and she finally sold her condominium. Kelly was ecstatic—until she found she'd gained 20 pounds in those two months. When Kelly came into my office, her eating was completely out of

control, and her newfound happiness was in a precarious state.

"Happy" overeaters such as Kelly feel very, very good and they want to binge on good feelings. Because the "happy overeater" enjoys food, she wants to eat as much as possible in order to fill up on these positive emotions. She sees happiness as a limited resource that will run out quickly and needs to be gobbled up before it disappears. It helps if she frequently affirms the unlimited abundance of happiness, since joy is our true and natural state of being:

"Happiness gushes forth from the centre of my being, bringing waves of joy throughout my mind, body, and soul, and bringing happiness to everyone who sees, talks with, or thinks of me."

Second, people with low self-esteem often feel that they don't deserve happiness or success. So, as soon as aspects of their lives—such as weight loss—start to turn out right, they unconsciously start to sabotage their own success. Happiness, if you've never had much of it, can seem scary because of its novelty. Even though it seems illogical to wish unhappiness on yourself, some people are uncomfortable with anything but morose, depressing days. They almost *need* a problem or crisis in their life to give them a sense of purpose. This is also an offshoot of Yo-Yo Diet Syndrome style number three—the Self-Esteem Eater, which is discussed in the next chapter.

If you're a "happy" overeater, it's important to remember that it really is okay to be happy and experience success!

Affirm often:

"My happiness is God's will for me. Happiness is my birthright, and my joy heals many lives."

In addition, the joy won't disappear or be yanked out of your hands, so relax and let go of any "lack mentality" that tells you that happiness is a finite resource. And most importantly, don't overeat because of your happiness.

9. Anxiety/nervousness

> Robin would overeat every time she was about to close a real estate deal. Brent found himself stuffing his mouth with food whenever he thought about asking a new girl out for a date. Heather ate bags of sunflower seeds before her midterms and final exams. Teresa felt as if she was starving when she learned she would have to appear on television to promote her company's new product line.

Anxiety and nervousness lead to a particular type of overeating—the "picking" variety. This style of eating disguises the amount of food one is eating because only a tiny amount is being consumed, bit by bit. But since the eating is continual, large amounts of food are eaten before the Yo-Yo Syndrome dieter even realizes what has happened. As if in a blackout or trance, the overeater seeks pacification from anxiety through food.

Those who overeat due to anxiety and nervousness use food to relax, so they need to find alternative methods to unwind. Since "anxiety eating" is so closely related to Stress Eating, people who eat as a result of this fattening feeling would benefit from following Step #1 for Stress Eaters, which is discussed in Chapter Seven.

10. Disappointment/hurt

> Elise felt hurt by the way her mother constantly criticized her. Almost daily, her mother would call and complain about

> Elise's choice of husband, job, and about how much weight Elise was gaining. In fact, Elise's mother always had something to say about Elise's body when she was growing up. These criticisms hurt Elise's feelings, and she regularly vowed to improve herself so her mum would finally be proud of her. But it seemed there was no pleasing her mother, and the more hurt Elise felt, the more she turned to food to feel better. The more she ate, the more weight she gained. And in this vicious cycle, the more Elise weighed, the more her mother pushed her to lose weight.

Similarly, people often overeat in the face of disappointment. Perhaps a friend lets you down or betrays you. Maybe you didn't get that raise or promotion at work. Or perhaps you feel let down every time you don't win the state lottery. Regardless of its source, disappointment can make you feel alone and hopeless about the future. It can make you lose interest in yourself, and make you not care what you weigh or what your body looks like. When you don't care, it's hard to stay away from food.

As with the other fattening feelings, methods for healing hurt and disappointment are described in Part Three of this book.

11. Emptiness/hollowness

> Terry had always let life dictate her choices for her. She went to a local trade school right out of college because she happened to read a newspaper ad for it. After graduation, she accepted the first job offer she received. Even though Terry didn't particularly like her new job—she didn't care for her new location, either—at least it was secure. To Terry, what mattered most was safety and security. But now that she had this security in her life, why did she feel so hollow inside? Why did she overeat cake, pastries or doughnuts every night?

> Terry felt that her life lacked meaning or purpose. My clients who, like Terry, have no sense of where their lives are going, all wrestle with discontentment, emptiness, and chronic anxiety. And these feelings all have the same source: not fulfilling one's "mission" in life.

I believe that we all have a drive or ambition to do certain things with our lives, and that we owe it to ourselves to try to fulfil those desires. We may not always succeed, but it's very important to at least try. Until we take steps toward our dreams and goals, an upsetting sense of uneasiness lives inside us. The goal could be anything from getting a high school diploma to graduating from medical school, writing that novel or volunteering at that convalescent hospital. Whatever your personal dream, go seize it! Break the big goal into smaller, more accessible goals, and then take one small step today to bring yourself closer to the life you want to lead. You'll be glad you did.

12. Grief

To discern whether unfinished grief could be at the heart of your Yo-Yo Diet Syndrome, ask yourself if thoughts about your losses bring about any of the following feelings:

- ☆ a heavy or pressured feeling in your chest
- ☆ tears in your eyes
- ☆ the desire to think about something else right away
- ☆ anger, resentment or depression.

If any of these feelings relate to you, you probably have some unfinished grief work to complete. Though not a pleasant task, spending some time focusing your thoughts on the pain of your loss (with a therapist, through prayerful meditation or by journal writing) could be the key to releasing you from your desire to overeat.

The most remarkable case I ever saw of unfinished grief work in a case of Yo-Yo Diet Syndrome was my patient Sally.

> Sally was a very pretty green-eyed brunette, but her 230 pounds were unhealthy for her 5′4″ stature. Sally had gained over 100 pounds since witnessing her mother's death when she was a teenager. Sally tried to erase the visual images she held of her mother's final moments by stuffing herself on high-fat items such as steak, buttered potatoes and salty junk foods.
>
> Our therapy consisted of reading letters that Sally's mother had once written her, and allowing Sally to simply cry, week after week during our sessions, over the fact that her mother had died. Once Sally completed her grief work, her excess weight fell off at a rapid and steady rate. By the time Sally was able to read one of her mother's letters and not shed tears, she had lost most of the weight and was no longer overeating.

13. Procrastination

Eating is, if nothing else, a very good time waster. It makes a wonderful excuse for putting off performing an unpleasant task.

> Ellen, for example, noticed that when she was ready to leave for job interviews, she'd suddenly get insatiably hungry. Her eating usually made her late for appointments with prospective employers, and as a result she'd avoid getting a job offer. The thought of going to work—and possibly being ridiculed, appearing stupid, or being fired—terrified Ellen. It was easier to stay home and eat.

Do you ever use food as an excuse to avoid doing some dreaded task? Do you use food to avoid making that phone call or writing that letter? To avoid doing a boring and mundane chore? To avoid completing a complicated or difficult task? If you answered yes to any of these questions, you've probably already recognized the futility of eating in order to procrastinate.

No matter how much food you eat, the task will still remain on your "to do" list. By eating before you tackle the chore, you only make things worse. It makes you feel out of control, fat, sloppy, and angry at yourself for eating. And you still have to face the dreaded situation.

Doesn't it make more sense, instead, to get the task over with (maybe even figuring out a way to enjoy it, too), delegate the task to someone else, or decide that you don't really need to do the chore after all?

14. Fear

Fear often triggers nervous behaviour, especially continual snacking.

> Needing some way to displace his pent-up energy, Ted spent the week before his knee surgery emptying the contents of his refrigerator and pantry. He was terrified of the impending surgery and general anaesthesia, worried that something would happen while he was unconscious. It was difficult for Ted to talk about his fears with others because he didn't want to appear weak. But underneath he was afraid. Very afraid. And his method for living with himself for that horribly long week before surgery was to eat as much as he could.

> Andrea was also a "fear" overeater, but for her, the fear was something she lived with constantly. Ever since she had been beaten and raped three years earlier, Andrea had felt jumpy and afraid that it would happen again. As a result, she overate snack foods. She munched all day long on candy, trail mix, nuts or pretzels—anything that was small and easy to pop into her mouth. The action of chewing on food helped her to feel less nervous and afraid somehow, but it also resulted in her gaining 40 pounds over those three years.

As we will discuss in Part Three of this book, fear is the root of guilt, insecurity and other fattening feelings. Although fear can feel like a giant foe, it actually has more bark than bite. By using the methods you'll soon read about, you can extinguish this unwelcome "guest" from your life permanently!

15. Boredom

> Time weighed heavily on Margaret each day. A 57-year-old grandmother of four, Margaret never had enough to keep her busy since her husband had passed away. So she spent her time baking cookies, cakes, and pies "just in case" company dropped by. But visitors rarely came, and Margaret would end up eating the desserts herself because she hated to waste food. When Margaret was finally able to admit that she actually baked the food for herself—not for her hypothetical company—she was forced to find other activities to fill her time.

Like people who eat out of procrastination, "boredom bingers" can fill up days, hours, months, and years a bite at a time. They're often anxious about having unstructured time and are constantly searching for something to do. They feel guilty if they're not engaged in some activity, and eating fits their definition of "activity."

If this description reminds you of yourself, it's important to come to terms with your underlying issues. Why isn't it okay to just do nothing once in a while? Do you always have to be productive to feel good about yourself? Are you trying to please someone or get their approval by staying busy? What other activity would you rather be engaged in besides eating? Why aren't you doing that other activity now? What steps can you take right now that will fill your life with meaning, purpose and fun?

16. Embarrassment

Colleen's husband, Larry, was an alcoholic who got quite obnoxious when he drank. He'd invariably embarrass Colleen when they were in public together by making crude remarks about her. "I just want to disappear when Larry starts saying those awful things!" Colleen cried. Instead of confronting Larry about his behaviour and alcoholism, Colleen would stuff her feelings of embarrassment and hurt with food. She'd eat huge portions at restaurants, and at parties she'd stand next to the snack table all evening, as if for protection.

Since a big part of Colleen's Yo-Yo Diet Syndrome involved her co-alcoholism (the emotional pain of having a loved one who's an alcoholic), her recovery necessitated involvement in the support group Al-Anon. This group, similar to Alcoholics Anonymous, is designed specifically to help family members cope with alcoholism. She learned how to be assertive with Larry, and she also discovered that his drinking was not her fault. "He had me convinced that he drank because I was fat," she said later. "Now I know that that was just his excuse. What a relief!"

Overeating due to embarrassment or self-consciousness occurs because of unrealistic expectations that you should never be noticed or be the topic of conversation. There is a tendency to take any remark as criticism, as well as a belief that other people's negative opinions about your behaviour are true. Then, if you do make a mistake—a social blunder or a business error, for instance—you feel as if the world's going to fall apart.

Intuition Integration for Emotion Eaters

As I wrote earlier, whenever you feel upset or hungry, contact your inner voice and spiritual support system! Remember that you are meant to feel happy and healthy, and emotional pain and an out-of-control appetite are signs that some part of your life is out of balance. Your intuition will guide you as to the best route to take to rebalance your life and return to a state of peace of mind and a normal appetite. During that moment when you think, "I can't stand this painful feeling. I must eat now!" or "I'm famished and feel absolutely drained and empty," stop and go to a quiet place where you can hear your intuitive voice.

Many Emotion Eaters ignore their intuition because they don't believe they are "strong" enough to endure life changes and challenges. They fear that if they follow the inner guidance to change their careers or love lives, they will face unbearable emotional burdens. This is a rational fear for Emotion Eaters, because emotional pain has accompanied many of their past endeavours. It's easier to remain in the status quo, believes the Emotion Eater, and ignore the intuitive urges to work on life improvements.

Emotion Eaters often carry years of resentment and grudges that clog their intuitive ears. You can unleash the full power and positive force of your intuition through a "forgiveness session". Based on the work of author John Randolph Price, here is a method that I prescribe for all my clients who are Emotion Eaters:

> Go to a room where you'll be alone and uninterrupted (put a "do not disturb" sign on the door and turn off the telephone ringer) for at least one hour. On one or more sheets of paper, write the name of every person or animal (living or deceased, personally known or unknown to you) who has ever irritated or infuriated you. Start with whatever name comes to mind, and keep going. You'll likely remember the names of people you haven't thought about in years. If you can't recall their names, but just their persona, write whatever descriptive phrase comes to mind (for example, "The head cheerleader with blonde hair from ninth grade"). Most people have a very long list, and usually their own name appears near the top. Next, say this phrase to each person on the list one by one (either mentally or aloud): *"I forgive you completely and release you now into the love that is the truth about us both. I only retain the part of our relationship that is healed and based in love. I ask that all effects from mistakes from the past be undone and forgotten forever in time."* Remember that you are forgiving the person, and not necessarily their actions (which are false illusions of the ego, no matter how hurtful they were). This forgiveness session will go further toward lightening your spirit and ultimately lightening your body than just about anything else you could do.

During the days following your session, you will see or dream about people who remind you of some names on your forgiveness list. This is no accident or coincidence, but is the Holy Spirit's way of showing you which persons you still hold grudges toward. As you get these reminders, keep saying the paragraph of release above, or pray for spiritual intervention to help you completely forgive. The more you release, the louder will be the voice of your intuition, and overwhelming desires to eat will reduce or even vanish.

Your intuition will guide you through every seeming problem you believe you have. You can tell the difference between your intuitive voice and the voice of the ego because the intuition is calm and loving, and the ego is abusive and anxious. For example, the intuition might say, "I believe I'd benefit from taking courses in yoga. I know the value of relaxing and honouring some quiet peace within, and I will now call the local yoga studio and follow through by attending the next class they offer."

The ego's spin on the same message would sound more like this: "Who has time for relaxation? If I don't keep busy, something awful is likely to happen to my job or marriage. Besides, I don't want Tom to think I'm worthless, and that's what he'd probably say if I did something selfish like taking a yoga class. He's so judgmental and unspiritual; he'd never understand why I took time away from the family to indulge myself!"

Decisions based on the ego voice rarely lead to happy outcomes. How does Tom act if you hold images of him as a judgmental or unspiritual being? How do you feel about yourself if you always have to look over your shoulder to guard against attacks by others? Judgments and resentment that the ego holds about other people always boomerang back to us as emotional pain. However, if you followed the intuitive voice, you would act in a loving way toward yourself and others. By focusing on the true loving and spiritual self of others, you invoke their true self to come shining through. Your life stays in harmony in this way, and you don't instigate situations that trigger emotional eating.

No longer will you cover up your intuition's voice with food! You have committed yourself to healing your appetite and weight, so today you fearlessly face the contents of your inner guide's message. Then you find that your intuition makes a lot of sense, and that it directs you to take steps that ultimately make your career, love life and health dreams come true. The more you follow your intuition, the more your life improves, your self-assurance increases and your hunger dissipates.

At this point during your Yo-Yo Diet Syndrome healing process, you may notice an increasing awareness of your eating behaviour. Some of the information you're reading may trigger some fattening feelings and may make you feel hungry for food. You may be, at this point, almost painfully aware that you don't eat because you are physically hungry. You eat because of emotional hunger. Understanding the reasons for overeating is an important step for Emotion Eaters. By becoming aware of the differences between physical and emotional hunger, your tendency to automatically eat due to fattening feelings will diminish.

Now remember to keep the 15-minute rule in mind at all times: the minute your mind veers toward thoughts of food and eating, note what time it is; for the next 15 minutes, don't go anywhere near food.

As I stated before, I'll be describing specific tools you can use to diminish and eliminate emotional hunger. For now, keep believing in yourself. You have so much power to make your dreams come true. *You can do it*!

CHAPTER SIX
THE SELF-ESTEEM EATERS

"The pleasures of the palate deal with us like the Egyptian thieves, who strangle those whom they embrace."

— Lucius Seneca (4 B.C. –A.D. 65), Roman philosopher

Style number three in the Yo-Yo Diet Syndrome is the Self-Esteem Eater. Here are the characteristics of this style of eating:

- ☆ Self-Esteem Eaters wish that they had more self-confidence.
- ☆ They tend to negatively compare themselves with other people. They are terrified of being judged, criticized or ridiculed.
- ☆ Just when the Self-Esteem Eater has lost enough weight to start receiving compliments or admiring glances, she tends to start putting the weight back on again.
- ☆ For the most part, Self-Esteem Eaters are motivated to lose weight to please their spouse, parent, lover or some person other than themselves.
- ☆ Self-Esteem Eaters have almost given up hope of ever losing their excess weight, and they wonder whether they are just meant to be overweight.

- ☆ Self-Esteem Eaters harshly judge themselves because of their excess weight. They feel like failures whenever they gain weight.

The metaphysical basis of self-esteem eating is a belief that "I don't deserve the happiness and orderliness that come from fulfilling my life purpose." Many Self-Esteem Eaters worry that perhaps they don't even *have* a life purpose! Other Self-Esteem Eaters lack faith in their abilities to succeed in their purpose, so they don't even try.

The affirmation for Self-Esteem Eaters is:

> *"I am created in God's perfect image and likeness. I am pure, powerful, holy, and very needed in this world. I have all the resources I need to fulfil my life purpose."*

Self-Esteem Eaters are those who don't feel very good about themselves and who overeat as a result. They lack confidence to leave or improve their unfulfilling jobs or unhappy marriages, and they're afraid to pursue their secret dreams and desires. The vicious cycle takes over when they overeat because they don't care about themselves. This leads to weight gain and subsequently to lower self-esteem, which means even more eating.

> Although she was a capable, competent accountant, Robin didn't feel good about herself as a person. The daughter of a depressed, unhappy mother, Robin was constantly told while growing up, "You'll never be pretty! Forget about getting a husband because you're too fat and plain-looking." Robin never doubted her mother's disparaging statements, and the 32-year-old blue-eyed, brown- haired woman truly believed she was ugly and unlovable.
>
> Evenings and weekends, Robin nibbled constantly, but she never thought of herself as an overeater. In fact, some-

times she wondered how she could eat "so little" and still be 85 pounds overweight. Robin was unaware of just how much she was eating, a nibble at a time. She was also completely unaware of why she was continually eating: to anesthetize her uneasy feelings about herself.

Here are some other examples of my clients who were Self-Esteem Eaters:

Painfully shy, Lonnie didn't have any close friends because she was afraid to approach people or initiate conversations with co-workers. She lived alone with a house cat and spent her free time holed up in her apartment with a book and a steady supply of snacks and meals.

When I first met Lonnie, she told me that she believed that others disliked her. "Nobody ever calls or comes over," she complained. Lonnie talked at length about how her "lousy personality" was to blame for her lack of friends. On and on, Lonnie expounded negatively about herself until it was clear that the person who disliked Lonnie most...was Lonnie. As such, she would punish herself by overeating and staying overweight. Lonnie, in other words, was punishing Lonnie.

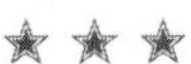

Jane, too, was a Self-Esteem Eater. A secretary for a law firm, Jane had a difficult time standing up for her rights because she was afraid to say no to her employer. She did favours for others even when she was exhausted and would have preferred to say, "I can't."

Jane acted like a doormat for the people around her because she didn't feel she had the right, or the courage, to assert herself. She soothed her wounded pride at the end of each day with a huge dinner and a rich dessert, a practice that kept Jane 20 pounds heavier than she cared to be.

Breaking the destructive cycle of Self-Esteem Eating seems tough because it means pulling yourself up by your bootstraps before you feel ready. Let me explain. Think for a moment about the people in your life whom you like best—the ones you'd prefer to spend time with (but not romantic interests, necessarily). Most likely, the individuals you come up with are those who treat you nicely and who make you feel good—people who you feel really like you, who say nice things to you, and who treat you with respect.

Well, this is natural, as we all like people who are nice to us. So what happens to us when *we* don't treat us nicely? How do we feel as people when we're inconsiderate to ourselves, when we allow others to walk on us or take advantage of us? The answer, of course, is that we don't like ourselves very much, just as we don't like *anyone* who mistreats us.

The ramifications of this condition, as mentioned a moment ago, is that Yo-Yo Syndrome dieters whose self-esteem is low don't feel that they deserve to be treated nicely. Although I spend a great deal of time helping such individuals increase their self-esteem levels, first I usually have to help new clients feel that they *deserve* to treat themselves well. Because they're so accustomed to kicking themselves and letting everybody else kick them, too, they don't know how to stop the cycle.

The paradox of all this is important to understand: before your self-esteem can increase, you must begin to treat yourself as well as you possibly can. This means you must begin taking good care of yourself *before* you feel ready to. You must be nice to yourself even though it feels selfish or makes you feel guilty. Then after a month or two of treating yourself so considerately, your self-esteem will begin to catch up with your new behaviour.

You'll start to believe that you deserve good treatment. Your self-esteem will be much higher at that point.

The section below lists several ways to increase your self-esteem and begin treating yourself better. For the Self-Esteem Eater, this step is extremely important in order to lose weight and keep it off.

Step #1 for Self-Esteem Eaters: Learning to Love Yourself

You really can like yourself before you've lost your excess weight. In fact, you need to if you're ever going to lose the weight permanently! And it's especially vital if you're ever going to allow yourself to enjoy the fruits of all your hard labour: a healthy, trim and attractive body that you yourself can appreciate.

Studies show that you need plenty of confidence in yourself in order to successfully lose weight. This is because you need to trust that you'll stick with an eating or exercise plan; without this belief, you'll end up saying, "What's the use?" and give up. Unless you like yourself, it's almost impossible to have any trust, faith or confidence in yourself.

If you haven't been good to yourself in a while, it's best to start with basic steps. The self-esteem exercises that follow are divided into two sections to be completed one at a time. I suggest that you spend at least two weeks on the first section and a month on the second.

Of course, taking good care of yourself isn't something that's just temporary. It's an endeavour you'll want to undertake for the rest of your life.

Section 1

This section begins with basic exercises that may feel like superficial indulgences at first. Believe me, they're far from trivial—

they're designed to set the stage for learning how to be good to yourself. While doing these exercises, you may feel guilty or foolish. If you do, don't try to stuff or ignore these feelings, but don't let them stop you from performing each exercise. Each step is important, so don't skip any of them—even though it may be tempting to do so. Remember that in return for your efforts, you'll get what you've always wanted: happiness, self-love and a healthier body. Does that sound impossible? If it does, then you really need these exercises badly!

Don't make the mistake of waiting until you're in the mood before beginning these steps. You'll never be in the mood until you start to feel better about yourself. In other words, higher self-esteem follows the behaviour; first you act "as if" you like yourself, then the actual liking of yourself follows. Start the following steps today.

1. *Replace Your Old Clothes.* Throw away or donate all your ugly clothes, including pyjamas and undergarments. Even if you were planning to wait until you were at that ideal weight before going clothes shopping, buy yourself some attractive new clothes this week. Buy clothing that fits you comfortably at your present weight—the nicest, most attractive clothes you can afford. Remember, you deserve them now! By putting off treating yourself well, you virtually guarantee that weight loss won't occur. You are affirming, through your behaviour, that your good is in the future—not in the here-and-now. Collect your "good," starting right this minute!

   As you recover from the Yo-Yo Diet Syndrome and find that you're losing weight, get rid of your too-big clothes as you go along. Then buy yourself more new clothes as you shrink out of each new size. Remember that by donating your clothes, you'll have a tax deduction, and you'll be helping people less fortunate than yourself. (Domestic violence shelters can always use donated clothing!)

You won't be wasting money by buying new clothes on your way down the weight scale. Just think about all the money you used to spend on huge meals, snacks, diet clubs, diet doctors and health problems related to your weight. Compared to all that money, these self-esteem steps won't cost all that much. And they'll give you the best return on your money that you've ever had!

Looking good now will help raise your self-confidence, make you feel better about yourself and also garner positive feedback from others. All of this reinforcement will make it much easier for you to lose weight because you'll get in the habit of taking better care of yourself—a habit that will naturally lead you to select foods that are good for you—and to stop stuffing yourself with food beyond the point of satiation. We naturally treat people we like with respect, and this will hold true with your own self, too, as you take better care of yourself.

Along with going to the trouble and expense of dressing well on your "weigh down" the scale, also remember to pay attention to your hair, skin, make-up, teeth, fingernails and other aspects of personal grooming and hygiene. If you need to see a dermatologist, make-up consultant, dentist, manicurist, speech therapist or other professional, make an appointment right away. Again, the cost will prove to be well worth it; think of it as an investment that will return multiple dividends.

2. *Treat Yourself Special.* Who would be the most special guest you could think of entertaining at your home? Would it be the president or first lady? A movie star? An author? What would you run out and buy, or what would you do differently, if you got a phone call right now tell-

ing you that this person was coming to your house for the weekend? Well, guess what? You're just as special. In fact, you're even more special because you live with yourself every day and not with the person you pictured above. Since you're so special, you deserve special treatment. Unfortunately, most Self-Esteem Eaters think in terms of settling for second best all the time. They do and buy for everyone but themselves, and then they wonder why they don't feel very good about themselves.

Stop settling for a second-rate life! If you'd do something special for the president's wife, then you can do it for yourself. But you don't have to spend a lot of money to treat yourself well. Here are some examples of small things that make a *big* difference in how you feel about yourself. Try one activity every day for a week, and notice how much better, more energized, and how much less hungry for food you feel:

☆ Get out your best china and crystal, and put away your plastic cups and stoneware dishes. You deserve to eat your meals on the finest dinnerware, and you'll feel special drinking your water out of elegant stemware.

☆ Don't always go to the bargain table or discount rack when you go shopping. While I'm the first to admit that getting a great buy can make you feel wonderful, it's also important to purchase something that's not on sale once in a while, too, if you really want it. Insisting on only buying sale items stems from a "lack mentality" that actually creates lack in your life. Paying full price affirms, "I have abundance," which is a mindset that inspires more prosperity to flow into your life.

☆ Treat yourself to a pedicure, massage or manicure (men, too!).

☆ Take a luxurious bubble bath, complete with lit candles all around you, flower petals in the water, your favourite music or reading material, and a crystal glass full of sparkling water.

☆ Keep a bouquet of fresh flowers in your home at all times. Just put it right in your grocery shopping cart instead of the fattening foods you used to buy.

☆ Buy new underwear. Believe it or not, the quality of your undergarments influences the way you feel about yourself.

☆ Ladies, please make sure that you have an adequate supply of pretty, well-fitting lingerie and underwear; and men, you deserve to have comfortable and attractive socks and briefs or shorts.

☆ Take yourself out on a date. Go to that new romantic comedy movie or action flick, spiritual workshop or ballet performance that you've been dying to attend (but that your family and friends seem uninterested in). Dress up a bit for the occasion, and treat yourself to some unbuttered popcorn!.

☆ Go away for a mini-vacation all by yourself now and then. This could mean checking into a hotel for the weekend, or house-sitting for a friend who's out of town. Go on a long drive to your favourite places, even if you say you don't like to be by yourself (as your self-esteem rises, you'll be more comfortable in your own company).

You decide what you want! You don't need anyone's permission to do something that's going to benefit you. Remember that your spouse and children will ultimately be better off if you are happier with yourself. Getting your needs met is up to *you*. And you deserve it.

3. *Get Emotional Support.* The need for emotional support during healing from the Yo-Yo Diet Syndrome is different for everyone. Some people find that they can't stick to the suggestions given in this book without another person cheering them on, while others say that they'd rather keep their entire healing process very private and maybe just discuss it with one or two close, supportive friends.

   Whatever your particular needs, I highly recommend that you attend a meeting of Overeaters Anonymous (OA) because it offers a warm, inviting means of support for Yo-Yo Syndrome dieters. People of all types—extremely obese to slightly overweight, young and old, men and women, educated and illiterate—find that the group offers a source of comfort and unconditional support.

   Each group has its own unique personality, so you might have to try more than one meeting to find one you're comfortable with. If you've tried OA in the past and decided it wasn't for you, you probably just weren't ready for it then, so you owe it to yourself to try the group again.

   Try at least three OA meetings before you decide. The times and locations are usually listed in the community bulletin board section of your local newspaper, or you can look up online to find the telephone number of your local office of OA or Alcoholics Anonymous (which often carries information about OA). The website address is www.oagb.org.uk.

Section 2

This section is best saved until after you've begun the steps in Section 1 and have incorporated them into your lifestyle for at least one week. Section 2 is also important for your recovery from the Yo-Yo Diet Syndrome, and you might devote at least one month to the steps outlined below. I really think you'll like them!

1. *Make Positive Affirmations.* For those of you who might be unfamiliar with them, positive affirmations are self-enhancing statements that you say or write over and over about yourself. You eventually incorporate these statements into your self-image and increase your self-esteem. They replace the negative self-talk you may have grown accustomed to engaging in, such as, "You can't do that; you'll always fail!" Such negative self-talk has equally negative effects on your daily life, because if you tell yourself you'll fail, then you're bound to do just that.

   I'd like you to make your own cassette tape of affirmations using the positive statements that follow. You may want to add some affirmations of your own, too. Just be sure they're phrased in a positive "can-do" way (for example, "I enjoy exercising regularly") as opposed to a negative phrasing ("I won't quit exercising"). Your own voice is the best one for the tape, because your unconscious will respond best to it. Read the statements calmly and lovingly two times each into a cassette.

   Then listen to the tape at least once a day for 30 days. At first, the statements may seem ridiculous or dishonest. That's okay—it's just a sign that your self-image is extremely negative right now. After just one week of listening to the tape daily, you'll find yourself becoming more able to accept the positive messages. At the end of a month, you'll truly believe them.

Our mind's ability to programme is extremely powerful! If you don't believe this, think about the way in which you memorize songs that are played over and over. Maybe you've had this experience: You're listening to the radio and all of a sudden a song comes on that you haven't heard in ten or 20 years, yet you still remember all the words to the song. That's because you programmed your brain through repeated exposure to the words years ago.

Affirmations work in the same way. Here are the statements to use, remembering to state each affirmation twice into the recorder. Leave a space of approximately five seconds between each affirmation so that later (when listening to the tape) you can repeat the affirmation to yourself:

- ☆ *I feel good about who I am.*
- ☆ *I am a lovable person, and others are attracted to me.*
- ☆ *I achieve success in whatever I do.*
- ☆ *I am good at sticking to and reaching my goals.*
- ☆ *I deserve to lose weight.*
- ☆ *I am honest with myself and with other people, too.*
- ☆ *I am a happy person.*
- ☆ *I have the right to change my life to suit my personal needs.*
- ☆ *It's okay for me to be good to myself.*
- ☆ *I deserve happiness.*
- ☆ *I deserve success.*
- ☆ *I deserve to have an attractive body.*
- ☆ *It is safe for me to be attractive.*
- ☆ *I am responsible for my own behaviour.*
- ☆ *I am responsible for what goes into my mouth.*
- ☆ *I choose to make myself happy.*
- ☆ *My friends are loving, successful people.*

- *I treat myself with respect and love.*
- *I take very good care of myself.*
- *I am comfortable asking for other people's assistance.*
- *I accept "good" graciously.*
- *I enjoy exercising.*
- *I like to have a fit body.*
- *I pursue my goals.*
- *Today, I'm taking steps toward a happier life.*
- *Everyone benefits when I'm happy.*
- *I am responsible for how I spend the moments of my life.*
- *I have the right to be happy and healthy.*
- *I can put myself first without feeling guilty.*
- *If I need something, it's okay to give it to myself.*
- *I can ask others for help.*
- *I enjoy losing weight.*
- *Feeling good about myself is more important than tasting food.*
- *I spend time in meaningful ways.*
- *My relationship with my family is better than ever.*
- *I love myself.*
- *Others love me, too.*
- *I am a valuable person.*
- *I forgive myself and look forward to the future.*
- *Others value me just for being who I am.*
- *All of my dreams are coming true.*
- *Today, I treat myself like a queen (or king).*
- *I deserve to be treated with respect and dignity.*
- *I expect others to accept me.*
- *I am open and honest.*
- *I have fun and allow myself to relax.*
- *I like to laugh.*
- *I am an interesting person.*
- *I deserve all the success life has to offer.*

- ☆ *What matters most is what I think about myself.*
- ☆ *I live my life according to my own beliefs and values.*
- ☆ *I love my body.*
- ☆ *I like being fit, trim and healthy.*
- ☆ *It's okay for me to be admired.*
- ☆ *It's okay for me to get compliments.*
- ☆ *It's okay to let others get close to me.*
- ☆ *I am a good person to get to know.*
- ☆ *Other people honour and appreciate who I truly am inside.*
- ☆ *I am a very special person.*
- ☆ *I am my own best friend.*
- ☆ *I like being with myself.*
- ☆ *It feels good to lose weight.*
- ☆ *The more I exercise, the more I like it.*
- ☆ *I listen to myself, and I trust myself.*
- ☆ *I have the right to express my honest feelings.*
- ☆ *My feelings are legitimate.*
- ☆ *It's okay for me to feel whatever I feel.*

If you have personal or career goals, be sure to add affirmations about them. For instance, someone who wanted to be a sculptor used this affirmation, "I am a successful artist," and a realtor created the affirmation, "I make $500,000 a year." Both persons made great strides in their respective careers, which they largely credit to their positive mental attitudes from listening to affirmations. These attitudes helped them believe in their abilities to make their dreams come true. And that belief in themselves made them take steps to realize their dreams—steps that may have been too frightening for them to take had they not believed in themselves.

Make your affirmations in the present tense, as if they were already true. By claiming them to be true now, you'll be more likely to act in such a way that they will come true very soon.

2. *Use Imagery.* Along with reprogramming your expectations of yourself through the use of affirmations, it's also important to visually reprogramme the way you see your body. I've found a definite correlation between the mental image one has of one's body and the success of any weight-loss programme. Clients who never get to their goal weight aren't necessarily suffering from any physical weight plateau. They just can't see themselves as thin people! Until you see yourself at your ideal weight, you probably won't attain it or maintain it.

   By seeing yourself as a thinner person, you begin acting like a thinner person. Thin people don't get trim bodies by eating huge amounts of food; they eat moderate portions of light fare. See yourself as if you've already attained your goal weight—instead of holding a mental image of yourself as a heavy person struggling to lose extra pounds. With the thin image, you'll feel more comfortable leaving food on your plate. You'll be more likely to choose low-calorie meals and eat them more slowly. You'll exercise more and take more time to groom yourself. And in doing so, you'll create the body that you see in your mind's eye.

   Many Yo-Yo Syndrome dieters feel, deep inside, that they *can't* lose weight, as if a thin body is something out of their reach. I've heard the following statement over and over: "I'm so much older now than the last time I was thin—what if I'm too old to lose weight?" Although an aging body tends to have a slower metabolism, its natural state (that is, having a normal weight) is the same as that of a young body. No matter what your age, you can lose weight in a healthful manner. *You can do it*, and you don't have to lose your sanity in the process with some forced, unnatural diet programme! But first you must believe in yourself, or you'll give up before the weight has a chance to come off.

To help you edit your mental picture of your body, cut out a magazine picture of someone who is similar to your "type" (that is, hair, eye color, height and age), and who has a body you consider attractive. Please don't cut out a photo of an ultrathin anorexic model, though. Your goal needs to be a healthy body weight, and many models are emaciated—not good role models for anyone. Keep the picture in your wallet, or tape it on your mirror or refrigerator. After a while, you may get so used to the picture that you don't even see it any longer, as if it's a piece of furniture. At that point, get a new picture to use.

You really can attain a healthy and fit body! Many people feel that they're somehow excluded from the "lucky circle" of folks who have attractive, trim bodies. They feel that they're biologically barred from slimness, and that the whole idea of weight loss is absurd. Such an attitude will always prove to be self-fulfilling, so beware of your own tendency to sabotage your weight-loss programme.

3. *Take Inventory.* Take some time to analyze your current life situation by answering the questions that follow. As a Self-Esteem Eater, your weight is a symptom of unhappiness, not the other way around. To lose weight, the underlying problems really do need to be resolved, but this can't occur unless you face the problematic areas of your life and do something about them.

Analyze Your Activities. Take seven sheets of paper and label one for every day of the week. Then number each sheet 1 through 24. This represents all the hours of the day, and each day of the week. Spend the next week recording how you spent each hour of the day. For example, on the Monday sheet you may write:

11 to7	sleeping
7 to 8	getting ready for work
8 to 9	driving to work
9 to 5	working
5 to 6	driving home from work
6 to 7	preparing and eating dinner
7 to 8	cleaning and helping kids with homework
8 to 9	watching TV and getting kids ready for bed
9 to 10	reading a novel
10 to 11	getting ready for bed

This exercise certainly takes time and effort to complete, but I found it to be extremely valuable when I first did it myself. After you're finished with your week (be sure to honestly fill in each hour), take a good look at it and ask yourself:

- ☆ Am I happy with how I spent my time this week?
- ☆ Were there any times I could have spent doing something different?
- ☆ What thoughts kept me from spending my time differently?
- ☆ What feelings kept me from spending my time differently?
- ☆ Did I do anything I didn't want to this week?

- ☆ If so, why?
- ☆ If I could have three wishes that would come true, what changes would I make in my life?
- ☆ What keeps me from making those changes (fear, insecurity, guilt, etc.)?
- ☆ How can I begin to restructure my life so that I'm happier with it?
- ☆ Is there some activity that I dream about doing, but am afraid to do?
- ☆ Can I break this dream down into easier-to-realize components?
- ☆ What step can—and will—I take *today* to make one of these components come to fruition?

Analyze Your Relationships. Next, begin to look at your relationships by answering these questions:

- ☆ Whom do I spend most of my time with?
- ☆ How would I describe our relationship?
- ☆ What part of our relationship would I like to improve?
- ☆ Am I negatively judging that person or myself in any way?
- ☆ Since negative judgments are self-fulfilling, am I willing to see that person and myself as loving beings in order to heal our relationship?
- ☆ Is there someone I would like to be spending more time with?
- ☆ What keeps me from being with that person?

- ☆ Am I afraid of certain persons?
- ☆ Do I guard against getting close to people? What am I afraid may happen if someone gets to know the real me?
- ☆ Is this a fear I choose to hang on to?
- ☆ Do I have the right to choose how I spend my time?
- ☆ If not, who does?
- ☆ Do I give people undue power over my life by constantly asking them for permission?
- ☆ Do I feel that I deserve to have healthy, happy relationships?
- ☆ Am I more comfortable in harmonious or in contentious relationships? (We are often most comfortable with what we're used to, even if it's negative.)
- ☆ Are there any feelings about my relationships that are affecting my eating habits and weight?

Now that you've analyzed how you spend your time and with whom the time is spent, it's time to focus on how you may want to change your activities and relationships in the future. After all, if you're not happy with how your time is spent now, how are you going to be happy in the future without making some changes in your life?

Analyze Your Intentions, Part 1. Ask yourself the following questions:

- ☆ Which people do I admire the most?
- ☆ What about them makes me admire them (for example, service to humanity, fame, talent, looks, creative works, income, lifestyle.)?

☆ What about me is most like these people?

☆ What would I have to do to live my life in a similar way?

Analyze Your Intentions, Part 2. Ask yourself the following questions:

☆ What activities (write down all of them, including weight-loss goals, things you'd like to buy, places you'd like to go, and intentions in the areas of education, career, finances, relationships and spirituality) would I like to do within one month? Within six months? Within one year?

☆ What do I see myself doing five years from now?

☆ Do I feel that I deserve such a life?

☆ If not, why not? (If you answered no, then be sure to listen to your affirmation tape as often as possible to reprogramme this negative belief. You definitely do deserve success but first you must believe it.)

☆ What steps can I take today toward my short- and long-term aspirations?

Analyze Your Intentions, Part 3. Brainstorm with yourself for just a minute and write down all of the different jobs, occupations, hobbies or avocations that you've ever admired or dreamed about (actor, lawyer, mountain climber, healer, psychologist, scuba diver, author, gymnast, artist, etc.). Make a list of about 25 different occupations and avocations that truly excite you. List only the activities that make your heart pound with joy just by thinking about them.

Look at the list for common links among all the occupations and avocations you listed. For instance, are they all activities that would allow you to change the world for the better and leave your mark? If so, then you probably have a burning desire to fulfil a meaningful life purpose.

Maybe all the activities involve helping others. Or, perhaps they're connected to making big money or reaping other financial rewards. Maybe they involve travel and exploring cultures of the world, or perhaps you're attracted to the entertainment industry, where you just know you could help move people in some way or lift their spirits with your talents.

Whatever the common link among the activities you've listed, it represents your own needs and values. If these needs aren't being met in your current occupation or lifestyle, then chances are you aren't satisfied.

Look again at your list. Are there one or two activities that especially appeal to you, that just seem to jump off the page because they seem so attractive? Circle these occupations or hobbies on your list (even if they seem like impossible dreams right now).

One more question: When you were a child, what did you want to be when you grew up? Why? What happened to that dream?

Seriously consider the following now that you've zeroed in on some dreams and desires: why not enrol at the earliest opportunity in a course that will train you for your desired occupation or avocation? If you're unsure where such courses are offered, then contact your local community college or parks and recreations department. Talk with your local college admissions counsellor. These folks are experts at matching people with educational and training facilities, regardless of whether you attend their institution or not. Also, public libraries usually have a section filled with college and university catalogues, and guides to accredited correspondence schools. Or explore the bookstores for information about career training and various hobbies. Hobby shops also offer wonderfully fun workshops to help you express your creative side and meet some artistic soulmates while you're at it.

Intuition Integration for Self-Esteem Eaters

Your intuition and angels are loving cheerleaders who constantly remind you of your true innocence and perfection. Whenever you start to think, "People who lose weight are genetically different from me. Why should I even try?" or "No one loves me. I'm so lonely, and food is my only comfort and friend," it's very important to take a deep breath and go within.

A major reason why Self-Esteem Eaters don't listen to their intuition is because they don't trust themselves. They put more stock in other people's opinions than in their own. I have found that many Self-Esteem Eaters have wonderful dreams and life goals, but they doubt their ability to successfully accomplish these plans. So they don't even try, and then they cover their disappointment with overeating. Many Self-Esteem Eaters are awaiting "permission" or encouragement to start working toward fulfilling their dreams.

Please know that God gave you a purpose that you are absolutely capable of fulfilling. Your intuition is a complete package of guidance that will give you directions one or two steps at a time. Much of your fear and doubt comes from looking too far down the road. Remember that all huge achievements consist of thousands of small steps. Focus on today, and ask your intuition, "What single small step can I take right now toward the accomplishment of my dream?" Then perform that step, and tomorrow ask for another set of instructions. Any pain you have about the people in your life exists only in your ego.

A great way for Self-Esteem Eaters to increase the strength and trust in their intuitive voice is by practising daily meditation and chakra balancing. My book, *"I'd Change My Life If I Had More Time"*, details ways to practise these important steps, as does my CD *Chakra Healing*. In addition, many metaphysical bookstores and adult learning centres offer courses on meditation and chakra work.

The benefits of these healthful practices include increased energy levels, feelings of wellbeing and consistent peace of mind. So many Self-Esteem Eaters feel tired and apathetic because of the incessant mental wars that take place within them—wars in which they believe other people are putting them down. These battles are exhausting and emotionally debilitating, and they also lead to overeating. You will notice these warlike thoughts when you begin to meditate, and it will take some practice to learn how to replace them with peaceful silence. But you *can* do it, and you *do* deserve the peace that comes from letting go of your ego thoughts of self-attack.

Meditation and chakra work greatly help Self-Esteem Eaters hear the intuitive guidance that will create successes in life. The more successes you have, the greater your belief in yourself will become. Your intuition will guide you through every aspect of your life.

Here's how to differentiate between the voice of your intuition and that of your ego: the former is like a loving friend or coach who boosts your confidence, while the latter uses scare tactics that rob you of self-confidence. The intuition might say something like, "I feel compelled to return to college and complete my education. I know this is a signal that my higher self is preparing me for new doors that are opening in my life. I trust and follow this guidance by calling my college counsellor now and making an appointment to discuss my enrolment for the next semester."

However, the ego would give you the same message in a much harsher way, such as, "Why did I drop out of college?

They'll never take me back now that I've been away for so long! Sure, I'd love to finish my degree, but how could I compete with all those students who are surely smarter than I am? Besides, everyone will laugh at me for being so much older than my classmates. It's too painful to even think about!"

When we listen to our ego, our actions and thoughts are tense and uncreative. Your ego wants you to ignore the intuition's urgings to prepare for a door that is about to open in your life. You would later regret this ego-based decision, which would further compound your low self-esteem. However, if you followed your intuitive voice, you would act in self-loving ways now that would prepare you for the future events that are built into your life purpose.

It may help you to keep in mind that your life purpose is for the good of many people, and that you—as all of us do—have a moral obligation to fulfil this mission. We each play vital roles in God's overall plan, and we need to trust that our Creator doesn't hand out these assignments haphazardly. Whatever your intuition lovingly urges you to do, *go for it* with full faith that Heaven will support you all the way.

You owe it to yourself to spend the moments of your life in ways that make you happy. And for Self-Esteem Eaters, it's a must when it comes to achieving permanent weight loss. My clients who make positive changes in their careers and social life always report a reduction in their appetite for food. By filling your life with activities that don't centre around eating, you'll think about food much less often. Your life becomes so full that you don't have time to eat as much food!

Please don't think that your responsibilities will go unfulfilled if you take some time to improve your life. Actually, the opposite occurs. When you make life-enhancing additions to your schedule, you are automatically rewarded with more energy and vitality. And since you can accomplish more when you have a great zeal for life, it's like getting a raise in the number of hours you have available each day.

★ ★ ★ ★ ★ ★

CHAPTER SEVEN
THE STRESS EATERS

"He who does not mind his belly will hardly mind anything else."

— Samuel Johnson (1709–1784), English author

Style number four in the Yo-Yo Diet Syndrome involves people who overeat when they feel like they're under the gun. Here are the primary characteristics of this eating style:

- ☆ Stress Eaters never seem to have enough time to eat right or exercise.
- ☆ The Stress Eater is so busy that some days she wonders if she'll drop from exhaustion.
- ☆ Stress Eaters feel that, although they are working harder than ever before, they seem to be accomplishing less and enjoying life less. They feel stuck, like they're spinning their wheels, with not much to show for all their time and effort.
- ☆ The Stress Eater feels that the only way she can unwind from her whirlwind schedule is by eating.

☆ Food and caffeinated beverages are favourite pick-me-ups when Stress Eaters are feeling drained but feel they have to keep going.

The metaphysical basis of stress eating is a belief that "I don't have enough time, money, or help to fulfil my purpose." Stress Eaters feel resentful that they have too many responsibilities, and insufficient appreciation and support to fulfil their life purpose. Stress Eaters also try to force things to happen, which results in frustration because their intense nature repels people and thwarts their goals.

The affirmation for Stress Eaters is:

> *"I release the need to struggle, suffer and procrastinate. I am happy to take complete responsibility for my actions and my schedule. I have unlimited resources for fulfilling my purpose. I expect, ask for and receive plenty of help from others."*

Stress Eaters' weights fluctuate as a barometer of how much pressure they're under at work and home. When their loads are light, so are their bodies. But when they start to feel stressed by deadlines, relationship problems or a too-tight schedule, then their appetites increase, leading to weight gain.

That stress is created mainly by two situations that I've seen over and over again in the lives of Stress Eaters. The first is feeling stuck or trapped in some area of life. The second is having an overworked lifestyle.

The Stress Eater must resolve the particular troublesome situation rather than attempt to ease the stress with food. Overeating, of course, only *adds* to your stress level, because it makes you feel fat, angry at yourself, unattractive and lethargic. This chapter will help you discover other alternatives to relieve stress.

Feeling Stuck, Feeling Fat

There are as many areas that people feel stuck in as there are people but, in general, Yo-Yo Syndrome dieters tend to get stuck in marital and occupational ruts more than in others.

Feeling Stuck in Marriages

> Jenny had been married to George, her second husband, for 12 years. "I knew before I married him that things between George and me weren't all that great," the 36-year-old nurse told me. "But I just kept hanging on, thinking things would change or get better soon."
>
> When Jenny related her unhappiness with her husband and described how he belittled and insulted her, she also explained that she was afraid to lose George's financial support if she were to divorce him. She was terrified that she'd lose the house and be unable to support her three young children. Although she worked and had her own moderate source of income, Jenny chose to stay in an unhealed marriage rather than risk a financially impoverished lifestyle.

Many women find themselves in Jenny's shoes, feeling helpless to do anything to change their situation. So they turn to the refrigerator or kitchen cupboard to temporarily mask their emotional pain. Women, of course, aren't the only ones who feel stuck in empty marriages. Men have their fair share as well. Many share a story similar to Ray's:

> A 40-year-old engineer, Ray had married his high-school sweetheart, Gloria, right after graduating from college. Ray was extremely devoted to her, and he put a lot of energy into trying to keep her happy—no easy task, as Ray found out during the course of his marriage.

> "I don't know what I'm doing wrong," Ray complained, "and I don't know what else I could possibly do to make her happy!" He described spending hundreds of dollars a month on Gloria's wardrobe and on dining out several times a week. "I really do everything I can think of, and I buy Gloria whatever she wants. But no matter what I do, she's never satisfied. All she does is complain about what a lousy husband I am and demand that I make more money to satisfy her needs."
>
> Ray found that the more frustrated he became with Gloria's insatiable appetite for clothes and other expensive endeavours, the more he'd turn to food to soothe his feelings of being an inadequate husband. Ray didn't want to divorce Gloria, but he wasn't happy with their relationship either. Feeling helpless to make the situation any better—"It's really been this way for 20 years. Why should it change now?"—Ray felt stuck, with no way out, a feeling that was putting ten pounds a year on his already overweight frame.

Often not trusting their own ability to make the right decision about their marriages, Stress Eaters stay in them for years hoping that things will somehow change for the better. They turn to food to deal with the powerful feelings experienced in such unhealed relationships. One client, married for the third time, told me that during each of her marriages she had gained over 30 pounds. "I realize that I ate during those marriages, as well as in this marriage, because I feel dead inside. Somehow, the food makes it all not seem so bad for a while."

I teach my clients to use prayer and spiritual healing to restore their relationships, as discussed in Chapter Two, as well as in my book "*I'd Change My Life If I Had More Time.*" Prayer heals every part of our life, including our occupations.

Feeling Stuck in Occupations

Donna was an attorney who wished that she'd never heard of the legal profession. Hating paperwork, debates and the pressure of deadlines, Donna was as mismatched as anyone could be for her line of work. In fact, the only thing that kept Donna in her profession was the huge salary it commanded from the law firm she worked for.

"I'm trapped, absolutely trapped," Donna complained to me. "Between the mortgage payments on my house, college tuition for my two kids, and putting food on the table, I need every dime I make. So how can I quit and start over in another profession?" Every morning, Donna would wake up with dread in her heart—dread over having to go to the office or to court one more time. She'd drag herself to work after eating a large breakfast, then she'd eat continually all day long. "It's the only way I can handle the pressure," Donna rationalized.

Another client, Jillian, had every confidence in her abilities to run the health club she owned, and make a lot of money in the process. The problem was that owning a successful gym wasn't making Jillian happy in the way she'd always dreamed it would. "It's kind of an empty feeling," Jillian told me, "considering all those years I've worked so hard to put this thing together. Now that I've reached my goal, I think, *Big deal!*" The anticlimactic emptiness she was expressing is normal in successful individuals who feel as if they've climbed the mountain and then wonder, "What's next?"

I've seen so many clients who felt stuck in their careers because an exaggerated need for job security made them ignore the fact that they hated the work they were doing. Al, for example, really wanted to become a hands-on healer, but he was afraid of disappointing his father. "Dad always tells me that my government job is the most secure position in the world. He says he's really proud of me for getting this nice, secure job. If I told him I wanted to quit in order to practise hands-on healing, he'd hit the roof!"

Another client, Kim, worked for an aerospace firm in the insurance department. "I really don't like the work I do," she told me. "It's boring, and my boss is impossible!"

"Why don't you look around for another job?" I inquired.

"Well, only 12 more years and I'll retire," was Kim's explanation.

Feeling Stuck in Other Life Areas

While most people feel stuck in their jobs or marriages, there are other areas that Stress Eaters often feel trapped in.

> For instance, 33-year-old Nicole said her mother tried to control her life, and she didn't know how to escape. Nicole's mother called at least once a day and lectured her daughter on eating, working, talking to people, and every other imaginable subject. "I'd love to tell her off," Nicole said, "but I'm afraid of what it would do to her health."

Eating to cover up a problem does not improve any situation, as most of us know; it merely gives us short-term relief when a long-term plan to rectify the situation is really what's called for. Are you stuck? If so, some of the questions below may help crystallize your thinking about the problem enough to help you form a plan of action—followed, of course, by the footwork necessary to carry the plan to fruition.

- ☆ In what areas of your life do you feel stuck?
- ☆ What parts of the situation make you want to change it?
- ☆ What parts of the situation do you consider positive, safe or comfortable?
- ☆ What frightens you about changing your situation?
- ☆ Are there steps you can take to improve your situation so that you won't want to leave?
- ☆ Is there a way of changing your outlook about the situation that will give you greater peace of mind?
- ☆ Are there steps you can take today (including changing your outlook) to help you improve or leave your unwanted situation?
- ☆ Are you, in any way, waiting for someone to give you permission to take these steps? If so, who? Why do you feel you need someone else's approval to change or improve your own life?
- ☆ How does feeling stuck affect your eating and your weight?

The Overworked Lifestyle

If your schedule is crammed full of too many things to do, and you never have enough time to get everything done, you may be experiencing the second major cause of stress: an overworked lifestyle. Stress arises as you rush from task to task, trying to beat the clock to get everything accomplished. If you suffer from such a lifestyle, you don't take enough time to care properly for yourself, you probably don't get enough rest or exercise, and your eating most likely consists of haphazard meals at fast-food restaurants. In addition, you probably reel from the momentum and don't know how to slow down your frantic pace. This makes you especially vulnerable to overeating, because you may use meals and snacks as an excuse to stop working for a while.

> My client Jennifer had an overworked lifestyle. The 33-year-old business owner spent most of each therapy session complaining about all the things she was expected to do at home and work: the paperwork and inventory control, the taxes and payroll, making sure her children got up on time each morning, and then dressing and feeding them breakfast before the school bus arrived. After work, she'd try to find time to play with her kids and help them with homework. Somewhere in between all this, Jennifer would fix dinner, and she and her husband, an attorney, would clean the house and get the kids bathed and into bed.
>
> After that, Jennifer would try to unwind by starting to eat an evening "snack" that normally lasted until "The Tonight Show" went off the air. When Jennifer first saw me about losing weight, she believed that she was a victim of a schedule that left her no choice but to run herself ragged and then overeat late at night.
>
> However, by examining the tasks that she had to perform, Jennifer saw clearly that she was doing them out of choice. She was the master-planner of her hectic days and evenings. Although she could readily afford to get help for herself—a bookkeeper for her business and a housecleaning service for her home—she hadn't given herself permission to do so. This realization was uncomfortable

for Jennifer to face, because it implied that she was responsible for creating and organizing how her time was spent; no outside entity was forcing her to do this or that.

Did Jennifer, after realizing her involvement in her overworked lifestyle, decide to live a simpler life? No—at least, not right away. Jennifer first looked at why she needed to stay busy and productive: She was afraid not to be. Working, regardless of whether that meant balancing her cheque book, sweeping the floor or managing the horticulture business she ran from her home, was how Jennifer defined herself. If she wasn't working, she felt somehow worthless. And guilty. As if she were bad.

Jennifer feared that if she slowed her pace at all, something horrible might happen. This vague fear involved worry that she'd be judged by others as lazy—a fear stemming from being raised by workaholic parents who pushed her to keep busy.

"The only time I got their attention was when I brought home straight As on my report card," Jennifer recalled with a tense expression on her face. "I remember this one time, I had all As, except for a B in math. My Dad took one look at that B and told me I should try harder next time. He didn't even say anything about all the As I had gotten in the other classes!"

With such high stakes—her parents' attention, approval and what felt like their love—riding on Jennifer's academic performance, the young girl began to feel as if she were loved for what she did, and not for who she was. She, like her parents, began to give herself conditional love. If she didn't do things perfectly, Jennifer would chastise herself. If she did things well, Jennifer would momentarily congratulate herself and then go right on to another project. By the time I met her at age 33, Jennifer's daily schedule was an endless list of back-to-back projects, errands and appointments. And even though she was a very accomplished young woman who owned her own business, Jennifer felt as if it weren't enough.

Enough for what? For the approval she craved from her mother and father. Reassurance from her father that he was proud of her. A hug from Mum to let Jennifer know she was appreciated as a person. And, most of all, the knowledge that both parents loved her and that she was a lovable person.

The Yo-Yo Diet Syndrome was difficult for Jennifer at first because it meant coming to terms with the knowledge that her parents' surface ego behaviours couldn't give her the love and approval she sought. Their true selves, of course, were pure love, and Jennifer would have to continually remind herself of the spiritual truth about the source of the love she sought. If she looked only to her parents' surface behaviours, she was depending upon an ego illusion to give her love. The ego—no matter whose ego it is—is incapable of giving or showing love. Jennifer realized that this didn't mean she was unworthy or unlovable (something she feared). It did mean, however, that Jennifer would have to provide her own love and approval by continually affirming that true love comes from The Creator.

Was Jennifer then able to let go of her overdone lifestyle? Well, no, not yet. She was still too scared to relinquish her hectic schedule, although she would tell me she wished she could let herself relax. Jennifer wasn't totally convinced yet that she'd profit from a more relaxed lifestyle.

The phone call came on a Monday morning. "Something's wrong! I need to see you right away." We scheduled an emergency session, and what I heard from

Jennifer was not surprising. She, like other Stress Eaters with overworked lifestyles, was finding that she was pushing herself much too hard, and her body was beginning to protest.

That morning she'd had a panic attack. Common among people who drive themselves past exhaustion, a panic attack involves a racing heart, waves of dizziness, light-headedness, an inability to catch one's breath—as if the lungs had holes in them—and a fear that one is dying, having a heart attack or going crazy. When I explained what had happened to Jennifer, she seemed relieved, but worried that it might happen again. "What do I do now?" she asked. Jennifer had finally hit bottom and was willing to learn how to relax.

After seeing a physician for a check-up, Jennifer took a week off from work. During that time, I asked Jennifer to compose a brutally honest list of her priorities. Once she'd done that, we looked at which activities Jennifer could cut out of her schedule. All those that diverted from her priorities were cut. Times for play and relaxation were scheduled in. Once Jennifer accepted that her health, including her weight, depended on a balanced, sane lifestyle ("After all, I won't get as much done if I die early," she told me), she let herself slow down.

Today, Jennifer is a different woman from the one I first met. She looks wonderful after losing the 30 extra pounds she carried from continual snacking, and her face has lost the tense lines and stern look it once had. But most of all, Jennifer is happy with herself today and no longer loves herself conditionally.

If the beginning of Jennifer's story sounds at all like your own, rest assured that you're not alone. Having an overworked lifestyle is a big part of being a Stress Eater, but it's also extremely difficult to give up. It feels frightening, as if you might lose some ground you've gained. Slowing down can seem tantamount to admitting you're weak and can't stand the pressure—as if you've failed before you've had a chance to prove yourself.

As mentioned before, though, slowing down doesn't mean decreasing productivity or avoiding worthwhile activities. Actually, it means increasing both while at the same time letting go of the hundreds of meaningless tasks that eat up your day and end up frustrating you. You know—those activities that leave you feeling resentful and empty after you perform them—the ones that make you want to eat.

Here's a phrase that you may want to post at your work area to remind you that you truly are in charge:

> *Time is not my enemy, and I am not a victim of time constraints. All pressure is self-imposed.*

Sometimes we feel controlled by outside forces that inflict their will upon us and rob us of all free time. But the truth is that we have said yes to everything we do in our lives. Sure, there are consequences to saying no, but it is always our choice to accept or deny any activity. All pressure is self-imposed.

In other instances, we fill our lives with chores, committees and activities to keep our schedules full. After all, free and unstructured time can make us feel anxious. So we sometimes tie up our calendar to give meaning and purpose to the hours of our day.

Busy schedules also prevent us from developing intimate relationships that might eventually hurt us emotionally. If you're always busy on a project, no one can get too close to you. So your busy-ness is actually a way of staying in control of your heart.

Some people get hooked on the adrenaline high connected to being in a crisis state. Adrenaline is highly addictive, and it's interesting that the word *rush* is synonymous for hurrying and the euphoria of adrenaline. Time urgency also makes us feel important and needed, and justifies us saying, "Out of my way, world! I've got an urgent matter to deal with here!" So, role overload can be physically and emotionally addictive.

The truth is that we have an abundant supply of time, and we are entirely free to do what we want with it. Every day, we receive 24 hours, free of charge. It is only our belief in victimhood that keeps us in any kind of victim role. We are our own time bandits. When we believe we are lacking in any way, we perpetuate the appearance of lack in our lives. Guard what you say and think about time. Instead of saying, "I don't have enough time," affirm that "There is plenty of time." Watch your energy level rise and your schedule open; this affirmation actually creates spaces for the accomplishment of all your priorities!

Our Energy Levels Are Key

When people say they don't have enough time, they often mean, "I don't have enough energy." Our physical habits do influence our body's energy levels. But even more important is our spiritual and emotional energy level. We dampen our spirits when we sell out or act unauthentically.

We sometimes get confused when we have a lot of tasks to complete. We wonder which one is more important and which one is low priority. Our true self, through intuition, guides us like a chain pulling a roller coaster along a winding track. Intuition is our ever-present counsellor for distinguishing between high- and low-priority activities. When we fight this guidance, we block ourselves and feel compromised. When we disobey or distrust our intuition, we suffer in our jobs and relationships. That is when our energy levels sink.

After a day of compromising ourselves on the job, we feel low. Our interactions with our children, spouses or dates don't feel satisfying. Our egos chime in with loud messages of self-blame, insecurity, anger or guilt. That's when we conclude, "I don't have enough love in my life," never realizing that it's our own doing.

We can't solve this problem by taking medication or by complaining about our lack of love. Those approaches only amplify the ego's voice and drown the volume of our intuition's loving guidance.

Meditation helps us hear and understand our true self's intuition. However, many of us—whether we meditate or not—are aware of what our gut feelings are. When people tell me that they can't hear their intuitive voice, I always say, "Yes, you can. You just don't want to hear what it is trying to tell you." They admit the truth of this statement, and confess that they don't trust the wisdom of their gut feelings. They fear poverty or being alone.

Step #1 for Stress Eaters: Evaluate and Reduce Stress

A good way to reschedule your day to allow for a more relaxed lifestyle yet still get the important things accomplished is to make a list of priorities. I highly recommend that you do so. On a sheet of paper, write down the five or ten things that you value most in life. These could be goals ("Finish my MBA degree by next year"), objectives ("Pay off the charge cards"), desires ("Feel better about myself"), values ("Spend more time playing with the children") or concerns ("Take better care of my health").

What is on your list is not as important as the *honesty* of your list. Many people are ashamed to admit, for example, that their family, health or religious beliefs are not at the top of their list. But if they aren't, they aren't, and that's how the list should be written. If it's a list written according to what you think "should" be on it, the list will be worthless because it won't be *your* list. Remember, also, that you don't need to show this list to anyone else.

After you list your priorities, write down the approximate number of hours you spend every week pursuing each one. For example, if you put "Finishing my degree" as your number-one priority, write down how many hours you spend in school and how many you spend studying each week. Then write the hours spent on the other priorities on your list.

After you finish, you may be surprised—or horrified—to find that you don't spend many hours on the things that are important to you. No wonder you feel frustrated—as if you're spinning your wheels and getting nowhere!

Your schedule, ideally, will show that the bulk of your time is spent on your first priority, followed by your second priority, and so forth. What's that you say? "Impossible?" Well, I've heard that before—and I've found that it's usually much more possible than people realize. It's just that they're not used to giving themselves permission to have a life full of activities they enjoy. Unfortunately, many people are like Jennifer—they have to hit bottom with their health before they decide to change their lives. But you certainly don't need to.

The following exercises may at first glance seem morbid or depressing, but they are designed to help you continue examining your priorities. My clients who've tried both exercises report that they're tremendously helpful in clarifying what's really important to them; in addition, these exercises motivate them to readjust their lives in order to live according to their priorities.

Exercise 1

Imagine that the phone rings and you answer it. It's your doctor with some distressing news: the results of your last physical exam are in, and your prognosis is grim. You have just three more months to live. During these last months of your life, you'll retain all your present physical capabilities, and you won't feel any signs of ill health. But at the end of three months, it'll all be over.

Stunned, you hang up the phone. What changes will you make in your life right now to enjoy and give meaning to your last three months? What's the first answer that pops into your head?

Of course, no one knows how much time each of us has left on earth; it could be one hour or many decades. Yet, most of us live as if we've got an eternity left. We procrastinate changing our lives, as if tomorrow—when that perfect moment comes—we'll get started on what we want to do. We act like children waiting for our parents to give us permission to live our own lives. And as a result, we end up putting up with unnecessary frustrations.

We often don't see that it's up to us to change things we don't like, because it's frightening to take responsibility for our own lives. Now ask yourself these questions:

- ☆ What changes did I think about during this exercise?
- ☆ How did I feel when thinking about taking the risk and making those changes?
- ☆ What keeps me from making those changes now?
- ☆ How is my eating affected by my feelings about my present lifestyle?

Exercise 2

Write your own obituary as you'd like it to appear in the newspaper upon your physical demise. Include in it all the accomplishments you'd someday like to achieve but, of course, write it in the past tense. For example:

> Jane Smith will be remembered as an entrepreneur who rose above incredible odds to build the successful chain of used-book stores known as "Smith Stories" across America. She spent her last years helping various charities build homes for the underprivileged by collecting many large donations. She also erected "The Jane Smith Library" in this town for use by handicapped children. She inspired many people to share in her charitable efforts through her weekly radio broadcast, "You Can Make a Difference." Jane was loved by many and will be missed by all.

While it may sound like a morbid project, writing your own obituary is extremely helpful in clarifying just what it is you want to get done in your short physical lifespan. Of course, no one enjoys thinking about his or her own physical mortality, but by being realistic in assessing approximately how much time you've got left in this life and figuring how long it will take you to achieve your goals, you can plan how wise or unwise it is to put off working toward them.

Many people fear being labelled "selfish" by spending money or time on self-improvement or leisure. Taking time from your family and friends and spending money to further your goals isn't selfish; it's merely a way for you to improve your life and the lives of those around you.

As a matter of fact, when Yo-Yo Syndrome dieters aren't happy with their lives, when they're living to please others and not themselves, they are particularly difficult to live with. The resentment and depression that spring from not liking yourself or your life rub off on your children, your spouse and other people who come into contact with you. A negative attitude can be contagious!

On the other hand, if you're happy and satisfied with your life, you'll be a pleasure to be around. You'll also be an inspiration to your children, teaching them values about life that will help them have happy adulthoods, too.

Now, is that being selfish?

It's important to understand what to do when you feel stuck or live an overworked lifestyle because both are intimately connected with overeating. You don't need to radically or impulsively change your life or slow your pace entirely. What you must do, however, is examine how you feel about your life and the way you spend your time. Be very honest with yourself during this assessment, and if you're truly dissatisfied, take one or two small steps to make your situation better.

It's also important to become acutely aware of how your eating ties in with your stress level. For Stress Eaters, like Emotion Eaters, the best way to gain awareness is through a journal. Make the time to keep a personal diary of how you feel before, during, and after eating. After keeping the journal for two weeks, look for patterns in your overeating by asking yourself:

- ☆ Do I eat more during the work week or on weekends?
- ☆ Is this tied in to feeling more stressed at home, or at work?
- ☆ Are there certain times of the day when I overeat? If the answer is yes, is this because I'm using food as a stress-management tool?
- ☆ Do I use food to procrastinate because I feel I've got too many things to do, or because I don't feel prepared or motivated to do the task in front of me?
- ☆ What are some alternative stress-management methods I would prefer to use, rather than food?

A Slimmer, More Relaxed Lifestyle

Stress is a symptom of a pressured lifestyle, one that involves worry mixed with both monotony and risk-taking. When you're stressed, you're living on the edge of your seat, taking a toll on your body—and on your weight and eating habits. Many people *enjoy* a hurried lifestyle—to them, it's not stressful to be juggling four projects at once. Instead, they find it stimulating and exciting. So stress is a subjective and personal state of being, and everyone's definition of it is different. As mentioned before, I've found that many Stress Eaters are reluctant to give up their stress-filled lifestyles.

For instance, 27-year-old Lynn had her sights set on an upper-management position at the firm where she worked. To try to get the promotion, Lynn worked overtime every day, volunteered to be on various company committees, and knocked herself out trying to get her superiors to notice her. In general, Lynn's life revolved around obtaining her goal.

When Lynn came to me for help with her Yo-Yo Diet Syndrome, it was clear to me that her overworked lifestyle played a big part in her eating habits. Every night, she'd unwind with a two-hour-long "snack", which Lynn justified by complaining that she was too keyed up after work to cook a normal dinner for herself. These snacks, as far as I could estimate, were adding an extra 1,000 to 1,500 calories to her daily total. So it was no wonder that Lynn constantly struggled with an extra 30 pounds.

When I suggested that we look for ways to loosen up her pressure-cooker lifestyle, however, Lynn immediately became defensive. "If I don't work this hard," she shot back, "I'll never make it to the vice presidency!" To Lynn, stress and success seemed one and the same: you could

> not get one without the other. Lynn was afraid not to be stressed, and she equated peace of mind with a mindset of lethargy or failure.
>
> We discussed business researchers' findings that the most successful people, including corporate CEOs, generally have attitudes that are sure-but-steady. These leaders inspire their employees with their genuine enthusiasm for the company's projects. Lynn saw how she had confused "enthusiasm" with a shooting-star method of job advancement. Sometimes we can try too hard for a goal and fail miserably because our own tension drives us—and everyone around us—crazy.
>
> Lynn agreed to experiment with a more easy-does-it attitude that would allow her to enjoy her job to a greater extent, while still staying focused on the brass ring. By giving herself some breathing room, Lynn found that her relationships at work became warmer and closer. Best of all, she wasn't so hungry in the evenings, and before she knew it, her excess weight had dropped off almost without effort!

Lynn's situation reminds me of what the great motivational speaker, Earl Nightingale, (co-founder of Nightingale–Conant audio-cassette publishers) once said: "We choose our work. It isn't forced upon us once we're independent adults. Doing it to the very best of our ability should bring us joy. If it doesn't, there's something wrong somewhere. It's very probable that we're in the wrong work or fail to see our work in the proper light."

Some Stress Eaters feel that their stress-filled lives aren't optional. One of my clients, 33-year-old Cassandra, told me that she feels guilty when she's not doing something around the house. She said that she didn't realize she could choose whether or not to have a stressful life—to her it seemed to be an externally mandated lifestyle. And ambitious Lynn, described above, was afraid she'd miss out on success if she relaxed at all. I reminded both of them that, truly, all pressure and stress is self-imposed. We decide on our stress levels through our mental outlook, by saying yes when we want to say no, and by making decisions about our jobs, relationships and other life areas out of guilt and fear—instead of out of love. Fortunately, if we don't like the results of our past choices, we can choose again.

Many people, fortunately, are discovering that it is possible to have a relaxing lifestyle and still derive the emotional, spiritual and material rewards they value from life. I've found that most Stress Eaters can add three dimensions to their lives and find an immediate reduction in their stress levels. The first is developing a trusting partnership with one's Higher Power, and turning the stressful situation over for spiritual intervention. This is discussed in Chapter Two.

The second stress-reducing dimension is spending more time outdoors. This has a soothing effect on overtired executives and office workers who spend so much time indoors and in cars.

The third dimension is increasing the amount of fun in Stress Eaters' lives, allowing them to break loose from the rigid structure that 9-to-5 (or later!) work lives are made of. Why not go to the park and swing on the swings? Or chase someone around the room and then tickle them? When was the last time you flew a kite or went to an amusement park or a comedy movie? What can you do today to add some fun to your life? Make this your motto: *Fun is a necessity, not a luxury!*

Stress is a part of life from time to time for all of us. And of course, not all stress is "bad"; it can be tremendously motivating. But one thing is true about stress for all Yo-Yo Syndrome dieters: if you feel pressured, rushed or stressed, please don't eat as a result. As you read the list below, you'll find alternatives to using food as an answer to your stress. You can also make your own list of food alternatives to keep handy (perhaps on the refrigerator door) when you want to eat due to stress. The list could spell out all those projects you've been wanting to get to but never seem to have the time for.

My Food-Alternative List

1. Write a letter to Mary.
2. Cut a fresh flower bouquet from the garden.
3. Paint my fingernails.
4. Call around to compare insurance rates.
5. Go shopping for a bookshelf.
6. Get a haircut.
7. Work on my embroidery project.
8. Organize my music collection.
9. Clean the fish aquarium.
10. Pray and meditate.

It's a good idea to include one or two pleasant activities on the food-alternative list. Use this list to divert your attention when your hunger pangs originate from your stress and not from your stomach. In this way, you'll feel good about spending your time in enjoyable, meaningful ways instead of overeating.

Other Choices to Make

In order to lose weight, Stress Eaters are basically left with two choices: they can de-stress their lives to reduce their overeating, or they can keep their lifestyles as they are and turn to a healthier method to control their stress levels.

The section above dealt with the first choice, but some Stress Eaters may not be ready to let go of areas in their lives that produce stress. For these folks, it's vital that they turn to something other than food to alleviate the turmoil and pressure triggered by a stuck or overdone lifestyle.

There are degrees of both healthful and unhealthful ways to deal with stress (other than eliminating the source of stress), as demonstrated by this chart:

WAYS TO DEAL WITH STRESS

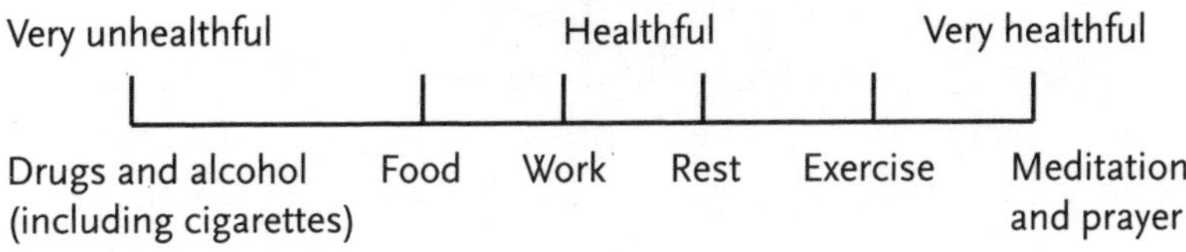

Drugs, alcohol, food and work are ineffective ways to combat stress, as most people are aware. Most of the time, these things compound and increase the stress level. People turn to them, of course, because they provide immediate short-term relief of stress and psychological pain. However, after these ephemeral feelings wear off, the stress returns.

Exercise, in contrast, is an extremely effective method of stress control. It not only helps to release pent-up anger and resentment, but it also helps build up resistance to future stress. People who exercise regularly find that they are less irritated by the small, irksome things in life than they were before they adopted an exercise programme.

If you're a Stress Eater, one of the best things you can do for yourself to reduce your stress level and your Stress Eating is to begin an exercise programme. This means exercising regularly four or five times a week minimum. I recommend that you exercise for at least 30 minutes at a time—45 minutes if you're up to it. The exercise can be anything you choose—jogging, brisk walking, tennis, rowing or aerobics—but it must elevate your heart rate to an aerobic level (see box below) and work your major muscle groups in order to effectively help you lose weight and reduce your stress level. If you're exercising and aren't perspiring, your workout is probably not sufficient.

Finding Your Target Heart Rate

Subtract your age from the number 220. The remainder is your "maximum heart rate"—the maximum number of beats per minute your heart should reach while you're exercising. Next, multiply the remainder by .70 if you have been sedentary and not exercised for the past six months on a regular basis. If you regularly exercise, then multiply the remainder by .75. This figure is your "target heart rate", the number of beats per minute you want your heart to beat when you're exercising.

To calculate your heart rate while exercising, find your pulse with the tips of your index and middle fingers placed either on your neck or the inside of your wrist. With a stopwatch or the second hand on a regular watch, count your pulse for six seconds, then multiply this figure by ten. This is the number of beats per minute, or your current heart rate.

If your heart rate, at any time, exceeds your target heart rate, slow down the pace of your exercising (never stop suddenly, however). If your heart rate is ten or more beats below your target heart rate, then speed up your pace or raise your arms above your head to increase your heart rate.

Many Stress Eaters find that stopping off at the gym on the way to or from work is the best way to fit exercise into their crammed schedules. Corinne, for instance, had tried going to the gym many times in the past but had always quit because it seemed so time-consuming. "I'd get home from work, and the last thing

I'd want to do was to change into my workout clothes and shoes and drive back across town to the gym. Now, I keep my gym clothes in my car and go right after work. That way, I have no excuse to avoid exercising."

Since most Stress Eaters turn to food at the end of their workday, exercising after work is an excellent way of avoiding the urge to eat. Corinne told me that she's inspired to keep healing her Yo-Yo Diet Syndrome when she goes to the gym and sees all the fit women working out around her. "I want to look as good as they do," Corinne says, "and I know I can if I exercise and stay away from snacking at night."

Melissa, another one of my clients who goes to the gym after work, told me that exercising helps her work off the upsetting feelings that build up in her stressful job as a customer service representative for a department store. "It's great!" she exclaimed. "While I'm riding on the stationary bike, I think about all the things that upset me during the day. With each pump on the bicycle, I can feel the anger draining out of my body."

Where previously, Melissa would take out her anger and stress on the food in her refrigerator, she now finds that exercising puts things into perspective for her. "By the time I leave the gym, whatever was bugging me seems small and insignificant," Melissa said.

If you don't have an exercise programme, take steps to begin one. Many people argue that they don't have time to go to a gym. In truth, those who exercise find that they actually have more time due to the increased energy that they feel from all the physical activity. They also have more time in their day because they spend less time eating and worrying. And after a month of regular workouts, most find that they enjoy (or at least, become accustomed to) exercising. Chapter Ten delves further into the subject of beginning a fitness routine.

Many well-designed studies show a link between aerobic-type exercise and increased production and levels of the neurotransmitter serotonin. Those who exercise, even moderately, enjoy increased serotonin levels immediately after a workout, which has several benefits for Stress Eaters. Stress and overworked lifestyles deplete serotonin supply and inhibit production. When serotonin is low, we feel groggy, cranky, hungover and jet-lagged. We also may feel hungry for carbohydrates such as breads, sweets or ice cream, since these foods trigger a boost in the serotonin supply. So exercise is a double benefit for Stress Eaters. Not only do you burn calories and fat, but you also ensure an adequate serotonin supply, so that your mood, energy level and appetite are balanced.[1]

The Art of Relaxation

Relaxation techniques such as meditation and yoga were once considered methods just for those who practised "alternative lifestyles". Now, scientific data shows that meditation significantly reduces physical symptoms of stress, including high blood pressure, laboured breathing and an increased heart rate. In fact, a recent study on longevity concluded that meditating twice a week is as effective as quitting smoking in increasing life expectancy.

Meditation is even more effective in extending life expectancy than exercise![2] The two methods together—exercise plus regular meditation—are ideal for Stress Eaters. Both will help you develop new habits for dealing with stress—habits that in the long run will end up reducing your stress level.

Probably the easiest ways to begin a meditation programme are to take a class or purchase a cassette tape with a title such as *Meditation, Self-Hypnosis* or *Progressive Relaxation.* Meditation classes are frequently offered through churches, community parks and recreation departments, adult schools, yoga studios and metaphysical bookstores. Relaxation CDs are available at most bookstores, especially metaphysical ones, or through my publisher, Hay House. I also describe morning and evening meditations in *"I'd Change My Life If I Had More Time"* in a script format that you could either read or make into an audiocassette.

I recommend that if you buy a meditation CD, choose an audible— as opposed to subliminal—voice track. While the music and sounds on subliminal CDs tend to be relaxing, the whole idea of subliminal learning is so controversial that I wouldn't even bother with it. Most studies show that voices and pictures must be consciously audible and visible before the information can be registered and stored in the memory. Any benefits you receive from subliminal materials, although real, are probably due to the placebo effect.

The main benefit of audible CDs is that they can teach you how to relax yourself by learning the methods of step-by-step muscle relaxation and guided imagery. Basically, these CDs will help you to slowly relax each muscle in your body, one by one; calm your mind and let go of worries; and create a soothing image in your mind, such as sitting on the beach watching a sunset.

Once you purchase the CD, it's important to actually use it. Many Stress Eaters buy a relaxation CD and then put it on the shelf after only a few uses. You'll need to schedule your meditation just as you do everything else in your life. If you feel that you don't have time to listen to your relaxation CD, consider buying a shorter one or rearranging your activities either late at night or in the early morning hours.

Take the time to relax...you've worked hard, and you deserve a break! And most importantly, the next time you feel hungry, wait 15 minutes to see if it isn't stress that's making you want to eat. If it *is* stress, remember that food is not an option for you to use in managing your stress. Exercise *is.* Listening to your relaxation material is, too. But eating is *not.*

Intuition Integration for Stress Eaters

Your intuition will guide you through every moment when you believe you want to overeat. During those hectic and stressful times when you say to yourself, "I must overeat," remember to think of and listen to your intuitive voice. You'll soon be bathed with an inner strength and serenity that will replace your tension and desire to overindulge.

It's important for Stress Eaters to get in touch with their intuition the instant they start to feel tense. By nipping your stress in the bud, you'll avoid a big build-up of anxiety that leads to unhealthful behaviours. The moment you feel out of peace, go within—you can even do this with your eyes open during business meetings or while driving, if necessary. Take one or two deep breaths, and release the tension-producing problem to the universe. Detach from the outcome of the situation for at least 60 seconds, and give yourself permission to trust that Divine order will solve everything beautifully. This moment of detachment usually leads to creative insights that were previously blocked by anxiety.

Sometimes Stress Eaters fear that following their inner guidance will lead to financial ruin or career disasters. Nothing could be further from the truth! Some Stress Eaters say they don't have, or don't want to make, time for intuitive introspection. While 20 minutes of meditation in the morning and the evening are certainly helpful for intuitive development, checking in with your inner voice doesn't require much time at all. I am not asking you to sit in a lotus position in your office and chant "om" in front of your boss. What I am asking for is that you be very honest and gentle with yourself throughout the day.

Your intuitive voice is always supportive and gentle, but the ego always acts as if the world is about to end. You can easily tell the difference between the intuition and the ego by looking to see if it's based in fear (the ego) or love (the intuition). As an example, the intuitive voice would say, "My corporation is about to be sold and go through a merger where my responsibilities will greatly increase, but not my compensation. Now would be a great time to follow up on that job lead I got at the networking meeting the other night." Notice the strength and positive phrasing, which are hallmarks of the intuitive voice.

Listen to the contrast when the ego delivers the same message: "Your boss can't stand you, you're about to lose your job; and you'll lose your home, your car, and you won't be able to face your kids. You're a notch away from being a bag lady!" If you follow your ego, your resulting decisions and actions will reflect its fear and tension. How could you make rational or creative decisions when you're terrified of financial ruin? However, if you listen to the intuitive voice, your job transition would feel safe, guided, and even miraculous or happily "coincidental".

The more you listen to and follow your intuition, the easier it becomes until you create a healthy habit. Just be careful of the Stress Eater tendency to force things to happen, because if you try too hard to hear your intuitive voice, you won't be able to hear it. Ask for spiritual help in assisting you to let go. Picture your mind becoming a beautiful open bowl, and visualize the intelligence of the Creator flowing into it. You may not yet trust other people, but you *can* trust the Divine order of this intelligence. Trust that this intelligence is always there for each of us, and know that it will supply you with all your answers. Breathe, listen, and take it easy.

Following your intuitive voice is your commitment to heal your appetite and weight—your declaration that, today, you fearlessly face the contents of your inner guide's message. You'll find that your intuition makes a lot of sense, and that it directs you to take steps that ultimately make your career, love life and health dreams come true. The more you follow your intuition, the more your life improves, your self-confidence increases, and your hunger dissipates. In the next chapter, we'll look at style number five in the Yo-Yo Diet Syndrome: the Snowball Effect Eaters, who find their portions growing larger and larger until they regain all their weight one more time.

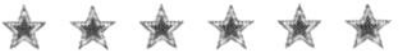

CHAPTER EIGHT
THE SNOWBALL EFFECT EATERS

"The appetite grows by eating."

— Francois Rabelais (1494–1553), French humanist

If you picture a snowball gathering momentum, speed, and size as it rolls down the side of a snowy mountain, you'll begin to get a feel for style number five in the Yo-Yo Diet Syndrome. This is the dieter who yo-yos because of food portions that grow in size, just like the rolling snowball. The Snowball Effect Eater's weight yo-yos because their motivation to exercise and eat less food yo-yos. Here are the main characteristics of this eating style:

- ☆ Snowball Effect Eaters' weights change during the seasons; they'll be one weight in the summer and a different weight during the winter.
- ☆ Eating is the Snowball Effect Eaters' favourite form of entertainment. They also view food as companionship. When they're lonely, Snowball Effect Eaters tend to nibble on whatever food is handy.
- ☆ Snowball Effect Eaters go on a diet because of some "crisis" (such as someone's remark about their weight or after seeing themselves in a family photo). As soon as the crisis blows over, their motivation for weight loss ends.

- ☆ The Snowball Effect Eater eats two or three servings of "diet", low-fat or low-calorie food, believing that "if it's dietetic food, I can eat as much as I want".

The metaphysical basis for snowball eating is indecision and worry about what one's life purpose is. The Snowball Effect Eater may seesaw between two or three different ideas of what her life purpose is all about. She frequently starts new projects and later discards them halfway through. Behind this indecision are fear and resistance to hearing the inner voice, and a deep worry that she will make the "wrong choice".

The affirmation for Snowball Effect Eaters is:

"I now quiet my mind and willingly hear and see the nature of my life purpose. It is safe for me to commit to that deep knowingness that guides me toward contributing to the world through my natural talents and interests. I now follow my intuition one step at a time, trusting that it safely leads me toward everything I want."

Phyllis was a Snowball Effect Eater who came to my clinic to get off the Yo-Yo Diet Syndrome cycle. She had been gaining and losing 15 to 25 pounds since she'd entered college ten years ago. The 28-year-old elementary school teacher had first put on weight as a college freshman, mostly because she overate to deal with the pressures of term papers and final exams and the overwhelming feeling of being 500 miles away from home.

Her first diet was given to her by the college nurse. "It was one of those hospital-based diet sheets," Phyllis remembered. "I followed it to the letter and ate exactly what the diet sheet told me to, which wasn't exactly easy considering I was eating all my meals at the college cafeteria." Phyllis rapidly shed the 20 pounds she'd gained, and after she was able to fit back into her old jeans, she quickly abandoned the diet.

The weight came back on in one semester, and Phyllis was horrified when she found, for the second time in her life, that she couldn't fit into her clothes. "So I went back to the college nurse and asked for another diet sheet," she explained. "But this time, the nurse recommended that I join a diet club since I hadn't been able to keep the weight off." And so she did.

The diet club, which met on campus, helped Phyllis commit herself to losing weight again. "The support was great," she recalled. "It was nice seeing that I wasn't the only one who was struggling to keep my grades up and my weight down." The club's recommended eating plan seemed easy for Phyllis to follow after her previous experiences with the stringent and bland hospital-based diet. This time, the weight took a little longer to come off, but Phyllis did lose the 20 pounds.

What happened after that was typical of Snowball Effect Eaters. "I was determined not to put the weight back on again, so I continued to follow the diet club's eating plan," Phyllis explained. She stopped going to the meetings and assumed that as long as she followed the same menus, her weight would no longer present a problem. Imagine her shock when, 6 months later, Phyllis found she'd regained not only the 20 pounds, but an additional 10 pounds on top of that!

By the time I met Phyllis, she'd been yo-yoing like this for ten years. Together, Phyllis and I examined her history of weight losses and gains and looked at each experience in detail until a clear pattern emerged. Phyllis would lose weight following diet programmes that spelled out specific 900 to 1,200 calorie and 20 to 25 per cent fat menus. She'd get in the habit of eating the breakfasts, lunches, and dinners in each diet until she'd lose her excess weight. At that point, Phyllis would continue following the diet but with one important difference: she'd become a "sloppy-portion eater". That is, she'd become inattentive in her portion control.

For example, if the diet told her to eat four ounces of lean skinless chicken, a plain baked potato and a mixed salad with diet dressing, Phyllis would follow the diet to the letter while shedding the excess weight. As soon as she'd reached her goal weight, though, the meal would look more like this: six ounces of chicken, a baked potato with butter, and a mixed salad with shredded cheese and ranch dressing. Within a few months, the "same" dinner would consist of a half a chicken with skin; a baked potato with butter and sour cream; and a heaping bowl of salad laden with cheese, pasta, croutons and blue-cheese dressing. Phyllis would increase her portions and condiments gradually and wouldn't notice how much she was deviating from the "core" meal her diet had specified—that is, she wouldn't notice until she had regained her excess weight.

Years ago, we believed that yo-yo dieting was the culprit behind successive weight gains. But, as discussed in Chapter One, new studies dispute this theory. Scientists say that former research that related yo-yoing to slow metabolisms was poorly constructed, thus producing invalid results. The only consistent data about compulsive overeating and binge eating point in the same direction: the psychological and emotional reasons that trigger overeating episodes.

Snowball Effect Varieties

Snowball Effect Eaters often gain weight because they mistakenly believe that once they are thin, they can eat whatever they want.

My 35-year-old client Pam, for example, had attained her goal weight after four months of following a diet she'd found in a woman's magazine. She assumed that the role of the diet was merely to help her lose weight. She never thought about making any permanent adjustments to her eating habits in order to maintain a steady body weight. "Now that I'm thin," Pam reasoned, "I can eat like a normal person again."

The only problem was that Pam based her idea of a "normal" person's eating habits on an abnormal conception. Pam's slender husband, Gary, and equally slim 14-year-old son, Tim, could eat whatever they wanted and not gain any weight. "I figured I'd eat whatever Gary and Tim ate," Pam explained. "Since they never gained any weight, I thought if I ate exactly the same as they did, I'd be as thin as they were."

So Pam ate as many fried pork chops, French fries and pieces of dessert as her husband and son did. If Gary ate a one-pound steak, so would Pam. If Tim had a stack of pancakes for breakfast, Pam would follow suit. Of course, it didn't take long for Pam to realize that her metabolism was much different from the rest of her family's—after she ended up regaining the 30 pounds she'd so diligently dieted away.

I call Snowball Effect Eaters such as Pam "backpedallers" because they remind me of cyclists who work so hard to ride their bicycles up a hill, only to abandon their efforts and goals by not pedalling any more. Backpedallers such as Pam slide right back into overeating.

Another Snowball Effect Eater, Jackie, a 42-year-old homemaker, had the same experience every time she dieted: she rapidly grew bored of what seemed to be one monotonous diet after another. "I can only take so much broiled fish before I start to scream!" Jackie told me. The longest period she'd ever been able to stick to a weight-loss programme was two months. After that, Jackie would go off the diet to eat what she called "real food".

Jackie was a "recreational eater", that is, she viewed eating in the same way that many see hobbies or vacations—it was her way of having fun. "I just love to eat!" she exclaimed. "There's nothing better on earth than a delicious meal."

Jackie's Yo-Yo Diet Syndrome plan necessitated her adding alternative, as well as healthier, forms of entertainment. Reluctantly at first, she joined a photography class as a way to have fun, get out of the house, and meet new friends. With the thrill of several successes in that venture, Jackie had the courage to sign up for a course in stained-glass making and another one in paper making.

These new activities created fun in Jackie's life, filled in her previously uneventful days with structure, and provided her with new friends and interesting things to do. As a result, Jackie found it easier to stick to her Yo-Yo Diet Syndrome plan.

I frequently receive letters from readers of my books who are recreational eaters. They plead with me to give them some secret method that will "let me lose weight without giving up the pleasure of eating". They literally want to have their cake and eat it too! I reply that, yes, eating is pleasurable. However, being overweight is both unhealthful and, for most people, not a very pleasurable condition. That's why it's so important to seek a healthier, no-food source of pleasure, such as human companionship, charitable giving or creative endeavours.

Another type of Snowball Effect Eater is the "seasonal eater". This is the person who gains weight only during certain seasons of the year—usually winter. Roxanne had no trouble shedding pounds during the spring, and she kept her figure looking great right up until the first autumn leaf fell. But right around October of each year, Roxanne's appetite would go out of control.

Seasonal eaters such as Roxanne fall prey to this phenomenon for various reasons. Some find that the cold winter months mean less physical activity and more time sitting indoors, thus leading to more opportunities to eat and fewer ways to burn off the calories. Others succumb to the pressures to eat that go hand-in-hand with Halloween, Christmas and New Year. After all, at what other time of year do you have four holidays that are so eating-intensive situated so close together—and focused on eating *fattening* foods, at that? Still other seasonal eaters feel that they lose motivation for dieting during the winter. For them, as soon as bathing-suit season is over, all reasons for wanting to be thin vanish as they cloak their heavier bodies in sweaters and wool skirts or pants.

Seasonal Affective Disorder (SAD) also compels some people to overeat and gain weight during the winter months. SAD is literally a withdrawal symptom from lack of full-spectrum lighting as the sun moves farther away from the earth during the winter. Two of the most prominent features of SAD are depression and cravings for carbohydrates, especially chocolate.

SAD appears to be tied into decreased production of serotonin. This chemical influences mood, and when not enough serotonin is created, the result is depression, fatigue and irritability. The body then signals that it needs help to produce serotonin, so it creates carbohydrate cravings for breads, sweets and chocolate. Carbohydrates boost the production of serotonin and also increase the blood sugar level. Both processes make you feel happier and more energetic.

Most SAD sufferers find that their appetite normalizes when they're exposed to full-spectrum lighting. For some, this means anxiously awaiting summertime. For extreme SAD sufferers with debilitating symptoms, a medical doctor usually prescribes a home system of special full-spectrum lights. The SAD sufferer spends a set amount of time in front of the lights, and the lights help the depression lift and the carbohydrate cravings lessen.

Still another variety in style number five of the Yo-Yo Diet Syndrome are the "sneak eaters". These people play a game with themselves while dieting, a kind of sleight-of-hand. The scenario of the sneak eater is often like that of Irma, who was constantly beginning, ending, or currently *on* a diet.

> Irma would always begin her diets with the best of intentions. "This time," she'd promise herself, "I'll follow the diet exactly." She'd diet down to within ten pounds of her goal weight, and then something would almost snap inside her. The 33-year-old receptionist would eat something that wasn't on her diet—a banana split or a package of doughnuts. It could have been anything, as long as it wasn't allowed on her diet. And always, Irma would feel deliciously wicked, as if she were being a naughty girl.
>
> The next day, Irma would anxiously step on her bathroom scale to assess the damages from her feast. And lo and behold, her weight would still be the same! Irma would glow with the warm satisfaction that she'd gotten away with her "cheating". This led her to plan other "cheats" that, unfortunately, got closer and closer together. Eventually, of course, Irma's continual consumption of high-calorie desserts caught up with her, and she regained the weight. Irma hadn't gotten away with anything but another cycle of feeling frustrated and fat.

One other variety of the Snowball Effect Eater is the "attention-shy eater"—someone who, when she loses weight, becomes afraid of being a thin person and eats more to escape back into the safety of her fat body. My client Betty was such a person.

> When I first met her, Betty complained that her dieting never took her below 150 pounds. No matter what she did, every time she got to 150 pounds, she'd go off her diet and start overeating again.
>
> Upon examination of Betty's pattern of weight losses and gains, I found that her plateaus weren't physical in origin—they were psychological. It turned out that at around 150 pounds, Betty's male co-workers would begin to pay sexual and romantic attention to her. They'd whistle and compliment her. One man even asked her out for a date. Betty, who was already struggling to keep her marriage intact, was afraid of her own reactions to all the male attention she got when she slimmed down. She felt flattered, but at the same time frightened (some of it was fear that she'd lose control and have an affair with her suitor). Betty's weight gains occurred because, unconsciously, she felt more at ease when she was overweight.

Then, too, there is the "apathy eater", who loses motivation while dieting. This was a real problem for Crystal, an attractive 35-year-old who had yo-yoed since she'd been a teenager.

> "The problem," Crystal explained to me, "is that half the time I just stop caring whether I'm fat or not. I always start my diet because I can't fit into my clothes any more, and I always tell myself that 'this time it will be different; this time I'll lose the whole 30 extra pounds'.
>
> "But it never fails!" Crystal shook her head and sighed deeply. "I'll get ten or 12 pounds off, and then I'll give up trying after that. I wish I could stay motivated to get those other 20 pounds off for once."

Step #1 for Snowball Effect Eaters: Get the Mindset

All Snowball Effect Eaters need one major ingredient in their lives to stop the up-and-down weight fluctuations of their Yo-Yo Syndromes: continual *motivation* to maintain a healthful eating and fitness lifestyle. Permanent weight-loss maintenance is a long-term goal, but it's difficult to keep the rewards of such an endeavour in mind when facing the immediate gratification from eating. The 30 tips below are designed to help Snowball Effect Eaters maintain the needed commitment, if not enthusiasm, necessary to heal the Yo-Yo Diet Syndrome.

1. Ask yourself: *why* am I trying to lose weight? Do I want to lose weight to please someone else (lover, spouse, parent, etc.), or do I want to slim down to please myself? These are extremely important questions, because the answers have a lot to do with how your diet will progress. Unless you're trying to lose weight to please yourself, it's going to be tough to keep your motivation level high. Do it for yourself, not someone else! After all, what's important is whether or not *you* are happy with yourself.

2. Get in the habit of weighing yourself every morning, right after you wake up and after you've urinated. In this way, you'll get continual feedback about how your eating and exercise habits are affecting your weight. The scale is simply an instrument to keep you from going into denial about any huge weight gains, since Yo-Yo Syndrome dieters often regain dozens of pounds without conscious awareness.

   Your weight will naturally fluctuate on a daily basis. It might even do so throughout the day from the weight of water retention that stems from eating salty foods, carbohydrates, or from your menstrual cycle. It's very important to use the scale as a tool, and not as a symbol of your self-image. DO NOT JUDGE YOURSELF OR THE QUALITY OF YOUR DAY, EITHER POSITIVELY OR NEGATIVELY, BY THE NUMBERS ON THE SCALE. You are not "bad" if you gain weight, and you're not "good" if you lose weight. Such judgments will put you into your ego state of mind, thus ensuring that you will feel emotional pain and that you will overeat in response to that pain. Remember to use the scale as a tool, and not as a moral compass.

Some scales measure body fat instead of body weight. Since muscle weighs more than fat, you may become fit without losing weight if you're working out with weight equipment. You may want to consider purchasing a body-fat measuring instrument (they aren't that expensive) and using it instead of a weight scale. In many ways, your body-fat percentage is a more important statistic to pay attention to than your body weight.

3. Write your goal weight (for example, 135 pounds, 155 pounds) or your goal body-fat percentage (that is, 15 percent) in bright ink on a large piece of paper, and hang it where you'll see it when you weigh yourself in the morning. That way, any discrepancy between the two numbers—the one on the scale and the one on the paper—will help keep you motivated to lose weight and body fat.

4. Stop thinking in terms of "diets" that have a beginning and an ending. Instead, when you begin the eating plan described in the next chapter, think of a total and permanent change in lifestyle and eating habits. A healthy, attractive body isn't something you achieve and then stop working on. Rather, permanent weight loss is a process instead of a goal to attain.

5. Related to this is the importance of positive thinking while you're slimming down. Instead of thinking that you're depriving yourself when you say no to fattening food, turn it into a positive thought by remembering that you're really saying yes to a fit, healthy body; and yes to feeling good about how you look.

6. Remember: "Nothing tastes as good as fit feels."

7. If you have a photograph of yourself at a weight you enjoyed, hang that picture on your refrigerator door. Try to find a picture that was taken when you were feeling especially good about yourself. When you get discouraged, this will remind you that you *can* get to your goal. Don't allow yourself to indulge in sentiments such as "Well, now I'm older, and I can't do it!"

8. Remember that your goal isn't to achieve a model-perfect body, but to achieve a level of fitness and energy that feels better than your present level. Focus on the *feeling* of fitness, not on its visual aesthetics.

9. The first three days of a light eating programme are usually uncomfortable no matter what you do, but once you get past the first day, the next day is easier, and the third day is easier than the second, and so on. Take it one day or one hour at a time, and simply concentrate on getting through *right now*. Don't worry that you may overeat tomorrow, because you can only control your eating right this minute. If you feel tempted to overeat, tell yourself, "Right this minute, I won't overeat. I won't overeat from now, 10:25, until one minute from now, 10:26." Then when 10:26 comes along, renegotiate with yourself.

10. Meal portions really are important! And since Snowball Effect Eaters are so good at fooling themselves about the ever-increasing size of their meals, it's vital that you stay brutally honest with yourself about how much you eat. For you, second helpings aren't even an option. When you eat something really tasty, make it last by savouring each bite. But don't go back for more until your next meal.

11. Snowball Effect Eaters must remind themselves of food's chief purpose: nourishment. No matter how good food tastes, there is no reason to eat more than it takes to give you a mild feeling of fullness. Admittedly, however, this is easier said than done. Those who have broken out of the Snowball Effect Eaters' cycle invariably follow these guidelines to avoid eating more than they need:

    - ☆ Chew slowly, putting your fork or spoon down between bites. This really works!
    - ☆ Pay attention to the taste and texture of the food in your mouth. Avoid reading, watching television, driving, or arguing with dining companions while you're eating.
    - ☆ These distractions take your focus off eating, leaving you unaware of how much you've consumed.
    - ☆ Notice your body when it signals that it's full (many people lose touch with this sensation).You've probably heard that it takes about 20 minutes for our brain to register a sense of fullness. A lot of calories can be consumed during those 20 minutes before you even realize how stuffed you feel.
    - ☆ Remember: This isn't your last meal, and no one is going to take your food away from you. Many people

eat as if there won't be enough food, or as if someone is going to whisk away their uneaten meal, so they stuff as much food in their mouths as fast as they can. Relax and take deep breaths between bites. If you watch thin people eat, you'll notice that they naturally take their time eating, or that they spend more time talking than they do eating. Here's something that is very effective: in the middle of the meal, excuse yourself from the table (cheerfully say, "I'll be right back"), go to another room, and stretch for a while before resuming your meal. This will give your stomach time to tell your brain that it's starting to fill up with food, as well as give you a moment to change your mind if you were just about to overeat. Try adopting these habits for a week, and see the positive results!

☆ As soon as you are mildly full (not stuffed), do something to officially signal an end to the meal, thus stopping your eating. Replace the I-must-clean-my-plate habit with a new habit of leaving at least one tablespoon or more of food on your plate. You can help your willpower to do this by putting your napkin, someone's cigarette butt, or some other unappetizing object on your plate. If possible, get up and throw the rest of the food on your plate into the garbage disposal. Then brush your teeth and floss (take a toothbrush with you to work and to restaurants), and find something to do to take your mind off eating.

12. Many of my clients have found that a good way to stop themselves from craving goodies is to use grotesque mental imagery. One client imagined that the cookies she was craving were made by hideous monsters with oozing sores on their hands. Another said she thought about

bugs crawling across the potato chips she was about to eat. This method is drastic, yet very powerful when your willpower feels low.

13. Pray. Saying grace is a wonderful way to add calmness and a sense of sacredness to your mealtime. Pray for Divine intervention in keeping you from overeating. Spiritual help is a powerful ally when you feel full of human weakness.

14. Yo-Yo Syndrome dieters need to create a pleasant ambiance during mealtimes. Instead of eating out of a can or a saucepan, instead of driving through that fast-food place and eating while you drive, make sure you sit down and eat your meal with attractive dinnerware and silverware. Put on some nice, soothing music instead of the upsetting evening news, and buy some fresh flowers for a centrepiece. A relaxing atmosphere will help keep you from gobbling your meals.

15. Along similar lines, it's important to eat your meals at approximately the same time every day. This helps set healthier eating habits.

16. Buy a non-food treat that you can give yourself the next time you feel like having a "goody". This can mean buying yourself a new CD or a book by your favourite author and saving it until you have a craving.

17. Don't put off exercising any longer. There's no better day than today to begin your fitness programme. Don't play that old "I'll wait until Monday" routine; you're just fooling yourself anyway. Some people spend their whole lives *planning* and not doing. Don't be like that with

your weight. Keep in mind this adage: "If it's going to be, it's up to me."

18. If you're a recreational eater and overeat mainly for the "fun" of it, then add some real entertainment to your life. Call your local parks and recreation department and see what classes are being offered—ballroom dancing, stand-up comedy instruction, photography, sailing, or whatever makes your heart sing—and then join one. Other ideas for fun: throw a "low-calorie party"—that is, one centred around something other than food (such as swimming, conversation or playing charades); rent a comedy movie; fly a kite; go roller-skating with a friend; attend a local theatrical production; go horseback riding; take nature photographs; take on a project such as renovating an old house for resale or rental; paint a free-form picture; or go to an amusement park.

19. Don't keep junk food around the house. If you have some in your refrigerator or pantry now, get rid of it. If this is impractical because of the needs of other family members, then make your own shelf in the pantry and the refrigerator. Remember that all foods not on your shelf are off-limits.

20. If you feel as if you're going to eat, go paint your fingernails right away! You can't eat when your nails are wet, and this will give you time to think about why you want to eat. Are you really hungry or just eating out of habit or emotional influences? Men can keep a pair of work gloves nearby to slip on when the "hungries" attack. Bulky gloves make eating difficult and nibbling almost impossible.

21. Visualize yourself in some outfit that you've always wanted to wear—perhaps a miniskirt, a bikini, a form-fitting outfit, shorts or straight-legged blue jeans. Make

the mental image as vivid as possible. The next time you want to overeat, switch off the thoughts about food by replacing them with your mental picture in your "fit" outfit. Picture the admiring glances you'll get from others, and how good you'll feel and how comfortable you'll be in your body. See yourself feeling safe and secure when experiencing this happy picture. Then ask yourself what you'd rather have—the food or the fit body.

22. Learn to spot your self-defeating thoughts about weight loss. Watch for those seductive little voices that tell you things like, "It won't hurt to go off my diet this week," or "Oh, what's the use, I've blown my diet today anyway."

    As soon as you recognize such a thought occurring, think about a tiny monster-like character and pretend it is he who is telling you to break your fitness vows. Give the creature a name and a personality; in other words, make this little monster an identifiable character in your mind.

    Then when you hear the monster's sabotaging voice, tell him (either aloud or in your mind) to "Stop! Stop that talk right this instant!" Picture the miniature monster running away in fright. The self-defeating thoughts should disappear along with your mental image of the monster.

23. Try to avoid social activities that revolve around food. Instead of meeting your friends for dinner at a restaurant, why not go to the park or go dancing together?

24. Reward yourself every time you have a day in which you honour your exercise and eating promises. Commit to paying yourself a set amount of money for each time you finish a workout or keep your meal portions light and healthy. The rewards of a new fitness programme aren't

always apparent in the first few days, and we all need some incentive for sticking with the plan. Spend the money on a present for yourself—something you normally wouldn't buy—such as a pretty wrapped soap, an accessory for your car, a new piece of jewellery or a coffee-table book.

Remember: you would have spent the money anyway, but probably on food. Most people tell me they'd spend any amount of money to stop yo-yoing. If this is true of you, then spend the money on non-food treats for yourself. Believe me, it's a good investment.

25. If you're a late-night snacker, then vow to yourself right now to make the kitchen out-of-bounds after dinner. Have someone else clear the dinner table for you, and bring any beverages you might want for the evening into the room where you'll be. Or put the beverages into a big ice chest and situate the chest in a barrier-like fashion in the kitchen entryway.

    It's a wonderful idea to take a walk immediately after dinner. This gets you out of the house (and away from food), helps you relax (so you're not as apt to Stress Eat), and burns calories. You might even make new friends or become better acquainted with your neighbours on your walks. If you feel unsafe walking around your neighbourhood in the evening, drive to an enclosed shopping mall and walk briskly around the interior walkways.

26. If you tend to nibble when you're cooking, be sure to keep a glass of water nearby, suck on a piece of low-calorie hard candy, or chew a piece of gum to stay away from the cheese you're grating or the sauce you're stirring.

    It's also helpful to write yourself a large note that reads: "Nibbled calories do count!" Put the card above the area where you prepare meals. You can reduce Stress

Eating during meal preparation by playing soft music in the kitchen.

27. Notes to yourself are really powerful. Write some encouraging words to yourself, and leave them around the house, pack them in your lunch bag or hang them on your wall. Cards saying "I can do it!" or "I'm looking great today!" or "I deserve to have a fit, attractive body" can keep you motivated.

28. Seasonal Eaters need to keep their wintertime fat patterns in mind as the first leaves of autumn turn. You can take control and undo this pattern, beginning this year. Reread these motivating suggestions every fall and winter, and then *use them*! It's such a wonderful feeling to wear the same-size clothes year round and not have to think of summer as a time to shed the winter pounds. I wouldn't trade that delicious feeling for any food in the world!

29. Avoid "all-you-can-eat" restaurants for at least the first month of your new fitness programme. Studies show that multicourse buffets trigger overeating in all animals, including us humans.[1] Snowball Effect Eaters are especially prone to losing all sense of portion control. The endless buffets at all-you-can-eat restaurants offer such a variety of textures and tastes that it's tempting to eat just a little bit of everything. This usually results in plates stuffed with food, however, and may send you back for second helpings of that food you especially enjoyed. So, if you decide to try an all-you-can-eat place after you've been on your new fitness programme for at least a month, stick to the following plan:

    Decide to eat only six items from the buffet. Walk through the buffet and decide, for example, on two different kinds of main dishes, two salads and two side dishes. Have only one serving of whatever you choose. No matter how much you're tempted to get "just a taste more", it's important that you don't. (This plan also works well for other kinds of gatherings where a lot of food is offered, such as Christmas dinners, weddings, parties, company picnics and family gatherings.)

30. Success begets success! When you see your body becoming fitter and firmer, you will feel more motivated to keep up your efforts. One simple way to speed up your success is by exercising for an extra 15 minutes each time you work out. For a small investment of a quarter of an hour, you'll notice a big difference in your fitness level right away.

Intuition Integration for Snowball Effect Eaters

Since consistent motivation is so important for Snowball Effect Eaters, it is doubly important for them to regularly check in with, and then follow, their intuition. If you are a Snowball Effect Eater, and you ever start to have thoughts such as, "What's the use? I'm hungry and I want to eat!" or "Exercise just isn't for me," stop whatever you are doing and take a moment to go within. Please don't wait until your motivation has sagged to the point where you don't care about your health, weight or fitness level. Ask for help the moment you feel your motivation waver—you can even do this when your faith and inner resolve feel non-existent.

Snowball Effect Eaters often resist going within because they fear hearing some awful news about themselves. I have found that many Snowball Effect Eaters have conflicted relationships with other people, and a major spiritual reason why these eaters lose their fitness confidence is because they don't feel good about themselves in relation to others.

Please know that any pain you have about the people in your life exists only in your ego. You can heal this pain! Your relationships can be very, very harmonious and loving—yes, even with those people you consider "impossible" or standoffish. Turn any judgments, resentments or grudges you hold about anyone (especially yourself) over to God. Feel the relief and the release as you lighten your spiritual and psychological load. Feel your commitment to self-care strengthen as you remember all the valid reasons why you're worthy of love and respect.

A great way for Snowball Effect Eaters to increase the strength of their intuitive voice is by creating and keeping a "Coincidence Journal". In a private notebook that only you will see, write at the top of the first page, "Today I intend to notice every coincidence that occurs in my life." Then, hold on to your seat, because many unexpected and pleasant occurrences will follow your written intention. You will find that the more you notice and write these instances down, the faster they will come into your life. Pretty soon, your Snowball Effect will consist of happy coincidences instead of overeating.

Your intuition will guide you through the seeming maze of all your personal and business relationships. If you ever get confused about whether you're hearing the voice of your intuition or that of your ego, look for the telltale distinguishing characteristics. The intuition sounds strong and reassuring. In contrast, the ego sounds either frightened or angry. As an example, the intuition would sound like this: "I feel that Sally has been quiet lately because of some personal problems she is having at home with her husband. I think I'll invite her to lunch. I won't pry, but I'll offer a compassionate ear and shoulder if she needs them." Note how loving and positive this sounds, which are key qualities of the intuition's guidance.

The ego's voice, filled with fear, would say: "That Sally is such a snob! She didn't even look at me when I said hello to her this morning. She must be jealous because of all the weight

I'm losing. Maybe all my friends will hate me if I keep losing weight!"

How would you treat Sally if you acted upon a belief that she was jealous of you? Might this belief propel you to overeat so you could gain weight in order to "regain" Sally's friendship? However, if you followed your intuitive voice, you would act in a loving way that would probably deepen your friendship and strengthen your own self-esteem.

By listening to your inner wisdom, your self-confidence and motivations for being fit and healthy will become strong and stable. The more you abide by your inner wisdom, the better you will feel about yourself, and it will feel natural to take good care of your body. No longer will your appetite and weight be determined by factors outside yourself. You will be guided by the source of positive growth for all areas of your life.

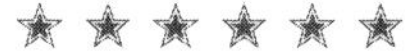

PART THREE

HEALING AND STABILIZING YOUR APPETITE AND WEIGHT

CHAPTER NINE

PRACTICAL GUIDANCE ON EATING RIGHT

"You will become as small as your controlling desire, as great as your dominant aspiration."

— James Allen, author of *As a Man Thinketh*

The above quotation by James Allen fits my belief that we must take charge of the contents of our thoughts. We can release obsessions with food, and we can heal overwhelming cravings and desires to eat! After all, we are powerful, unlimited beings created in the image and likeness of the Divine Almighty. We deserve to have wondrous aspirations that propel our imaginations and energy to the highest of heights. We are stronger than a box of cookies!

Fuelling the Body

The psychological and spiritual principles in this book can be used in conjunction with any weight-reduction eating plan. However, I'm often asked for recommendations about "what to eat", so I want to outline some general recommendations.

The thrust of breaking the Yo-Yo Diet Syndrome is to enable you to lose weight and maintain that weight loss by avoiding emotion- and stress-induced overeating. This means stabilizing your moods, and being able to recognize and quickly replace the negative thoughts that produce unpleasant moods. I am also recommending ways to uncover the intuitive voice that may frighten you into covering it up with food.

To attain these goals, you'll eat in ways that maximize your concentration and intuitive powers, while also helping your energy stay at optimum levels. First, here are four general guidelines about eating:

Guideline 1: Always Eat Three Meals a Day

It's important to eat three times a day, although I understand that this concept makes some people anxious. "But I'll gain weight if I do that!" you may be saying right now. I used to believe that if I ate breakfast, I'd gain weight—never realizing that skipping breakfast was keeping me 10 to 55 pounds heavier than I wanted to be. Many of my patients listen to my advice about yo-yo dieting under protest, insisting, "It'll make me fat to eat three times a day!" But they try it because others have lost weight at my clinics.

These clients are astonished to watch their weight drop without starving themselves, taking diet pills or buying special foods—just as I was when I first discovered this "secret".

If you skip breakfast, you've probably noticed that you don't get hungry in the early afternoon. Many people conclude that eating breakfast makes them hungrier and therefore makes them eat more food. However, the reason you feel hungry a couple of hours after eating breakfast is that your metabolism—the process that makes you burn calories—has sped up. If you skip breakfast, your metabolism slows down. Therefore, if you skip breakfast, you'll have great difficulty losing weight permanently.

Breakfast is also important because, without it, your blood sugar level drops, leading to low energy levels and depression. These feelings of fatigue can bring on food binges later in the day as you try to "medicate" the sleepy feelings with food.

Skipping meals does not erase calories from previous binges. The only thing it does is slow down your metabolism so calories take longer to burn. A sluggish metabolism does not "undo" the chocolate cake eaten the day before.

Skipping meals also sets you up to overeat at your next meal. If you skip breakfast, lunch or dinner, your blood sugar level will drop, and you will probably feel light-headed, irritable and weak. Under these conditions, you will be less likely to have the presence of mind to avoid your binge foods at the next meal. When you don't feel well, you are also less likely to *care* whether you lose weight or not.

Make sure you always eat three meals per day, and never skip a meal! Some people approach eating in a way I call "creative dieting". Through this process, a person uses various rationales for skipping meals, such as: "I ate that big dinner and fattening dessert last night, so I'll skip breakfast this morning." Creative dieters approach eating much like the person who juggles money and floats cheques to avoid bouncing checks. The juggling system doesn't work very well with either eating or money because it usually ends up collapsing on itself.

If you're a creative dieter, consider this thought for a moment: if you knew you had to eat three meals a day, would you be as likely to eat a huge dinner or dessert? Or does your creative approach to dieting give you implied "permission" to binge on fattening foods? If it does, then you have fallen into a common, but erroneous, approach to weight loss. One final question that creative dieters might ask themselves is: "If my creative dieting system worked, would I need to lose weight today?"

Guideline 2: Plan Your Meals Before You Eat Them

Most Yo-Yo Syndrome dieters eat in inconsistent, haphazard ways. I know that I used to! I'd wait until shortly before dinnertime to think about what I was going to eat, and then I'd go to the grocery store practically every day to shop for that day's meals (which is a time-wasting, expensive and fattening habit common to many Yo-Yo Syndrome dieters).

Planning your meals helps you lose weight for two reasons. First, if you plan what you're going to eat, you reduce your chances of overeating whatever is in your refrigerator or pantry. How many times have you come home from work, felt as though you were starving, and impatiently ate whatever was handy? If you plan for this normal reaction by having dinner ready at an earlier time, you won't have to overeat in the late afternoon.

Second, going to the grocery store for dinner at the last minute increases the likelihood that you'll head for fattening, processed foods. Most people know that shopping on an empty stomach is not a good idea, but they do it anyway. In fact, some people overeat *before* going to the store because they rationalize that they're not supposed to shop on an empty stomach.

Consider coming up with 14 days' worth of low-fat dinner menus. Choose your menus from low-fat cookbooks and speciality magazines. Stick to this 14-day menu, and shop in accordance with it. Your family won't get bored, because you'll only repeat each meal twice within the month. Of course, you can always add in new recipes as you discover them. By developing a plan, you'll eliminate that "What should I fix for dinner?" quandary from your life forever!

Guideline 3: Eat Only One Helping

No matter how tempted you are to go back for another taste, more salad dressing, or a second serving, DON'T DO IT. Make this a very strict guideline in your mind, especially if you're a Snowball Effect Eater.

As we've discussed, portion control is essential to losing weight and maintaining that weight loss. The easiest way to ensure that your portions stay light is by eliminating second helpings altogether.

When you eat lighter, it is much easier to concentrate and focus during meditation. Those who have honed their psychic abilities find that light eating contributes to increased clairvoyance. Heavy meals weigh down both the body and the spirit, while lighter meals have the opposite effect.

By adopting a black-and-white policy about the number of servings you eat, you'll lose the habit of debating with yourself. You probably know the words to this oft-heard refrain well: "That tasted so good, I think I'll have more. But I can't because I'm trying to lose weight. Just a little bit more can't hurt. I shouldn't. I want to!" These internal arguments invariably end with an impulsive rush to have a second or third helping before you have a chance to change your mind.

Just think of the peace of mind that comes from eliminating all ambiguity about second and third helpings. You'll eventually develop a habitual thinking process that goes something like this: "That sure tasted good, and I'd love to have another helping. But I don't have seconds, so it's not an option. I'll just wait until my next meal to have more of that food." You can keep your mind off second helpings by brushing your teeth right after a meal, and by immediately diving into a meaningful activity.

Guideline 4: Cook and Eat with Love

We eat less food and digest our meals more easily when our mealtimes are tranquil and love-filled. This starts with meal preparation. If you're the one cooking the meal and you're rushed, are in a bad mood or you feel resentful because the family isn't helping you, stop before entering the kitchen. Your bad mood will be absorbed by the food you're about to prepare. So close your eyes and take a deep breath. Say a prayer for strength and deliverance from your negative feelings. Identify and replace the negative thought triggering your unpleasant feelings. Affirm: "This moment is filled with love right now."

I strongly believe that we mustn't ever force ourselves to do anything we don't want to do. Instead, we need to take the time to rearrange our thoughts so that we either decide to say no to the task or feel love for the moment in which we are completing it. We really can make every moment a blessing. So when cooking a meal, look for ways to enrich the experience: play beautiful music or an interesting audio book, think loving thoughts, or look out the window at a beautiful nature scene. Whatever brings love into your heart, do that activity while preparing your meals.

Along the same lines, use caution when eating foods prepared by unloving hands. If you walk into a restaurant or fast-food establishment, for example, and you hear the cooks arguing or you can see that the employees are miserable, I would recommend leaving. If you do eat there, bless your food with love to transmute the cooks' negativity from the meal.

A rushed, harried meal creates negative feelings, stress, and even illness. You can add ambiance and a peaceful atmosphere to your meals by saying grace or a prayer of gratitude, turning off the television or negative radio talk shows, lighting candles, playing soft music in the background, and having a rigorous "no arguments at the dinner table" family policy.

Food Guidelines

What types of foods are recommended? As I've mentioned previously, when taking steps to heal yourself from the Yo-Yo Diet Syndrome, there are no "good" or "bad" foods. What is important is for you to decide why you want a certain food, and once you eat it, to decide how that food makes you feel. If the food interferes with your mood stability or your ability to concentrate or meditate, *then the food is fattening for you.* By eliminating that food from your menus, your weight loss will naturally follow—

not only because your calories are reduced, but also because your body and mind will be operating at their natural, optimum levels. So you will need to experiment, and eliminate foods if you experience any adverse reactions to them.

In general, though, light and natural foods are associated with the type of tranquil concentration abilities that will help you feel great and be in touch with your intuitive self throughout each day. You really will feel different eating a diet rich in vegetables, fruits and wholegrain bread products. Organic foods, too, seem to carry an almost etheric quality that translates into better feelings upon eating them. I've always believed that part of this effect comes from the love that people who work on organic farms put into their jobs.

During my meditations, I've asked what I could do to increase my intuitive awareness and powers. Every time I would ask this question, I saw the same picture in my mind's eye: chicken meat. Finally, after seeing this picture for the fifth time, I asked my inner guide why I was seeing this unappetizing sight. My intuitive voice told me that when I ate poultry (at the time I wasn't eating any red meat), I was literally ingesting the pain that the chicken or turkey had felt upon its death. My inner guide told me that the pain permeated the fowl's body, and that the consumed pain was blocking the complete opening of my full intuitive abilities.

Could this be true, I wondered, in semi-disbelief? I called a friend of mine who is an experienced spiritual healer and teacher, and he confirmed that he'd come to the same conclusion years ago. That's why he's a vegetarian, he explained. He said that it's common for people who are new to meditation to first give up red meat, then poultry, then seafood. Well, I've given up fowl, but at this point, I have no "messages" from my inner guide that I should stop eating fish.

In the meantime, I've discovered the whole world of vegetarian burgers, chicken-like patties, and even vegetable patties that taste and feel like steak. These are available in the freezer section of health-food stores and many major supermarkets. Even my very picky teenage son and my not-so-picky husband love these vegetarian meat substitutes. Vegetable patties are very easy to cook, and they make excellent substitutes for dishes calling for hamburger or chicken.

A semi-vegetarian or vegetarian diet is perfect for Yo-Yo Syndrome dieters because it aids in keeping your mood tranquil, your energy level stable and your focus sharp. Vegetarian meals automatically eliminate the saturated fat and calories contained in meat and fowl (unless you use a lot of cheese and high-fat sauces).

In short, if you follow the Four Meal Guidelines: (1) always eat three meals a day; (2) plan your meals before you eat them; (3) eat only one helping; (4) cook and eat with love; and if you also adopt a lighter, more vegetarian menu, and avoid emotion- or stress-induced eating, your weight loss will naturally follow. You can increase your weight-loss rate by adopting a regular exercise programme. You don't have to struggle or beat yourself up in order to lose weight! Use these meal guidelines and find how peaceful weight loss and maintenance can be.

Other Guidelines: Between-Meal Snacks

Some people who suffer from the Yo-Yo Diet Syndrome don't know how to snack. For example, a well-intentioned snack may start off with a cracker and the rationalization that "it only has ten calories". This sets off a craving for another cracker, but this time topped with cheese because "I have to have protein in my diet." One cracker-with-cheese is followed by another and another until the "snack" gains momentum and turns into a full-blown eating binge. The snack becomes an endless food bridge connecting breakfast to lunch to dinner.

If this sounds like you, then you may be someone who cannot snack. In other words, some people have a propensity to do things in an all-or-nothing way and cannot do anything in moderation. For these folks, there's no such thing as a "snack" or a small treat. Every time they eat between meals, they keep munching away. To combat this natural tendency to eat without stop, you can either ensure that your snacks are ultra-low calorie (such as carrot sticks, broccoli florets, celery, unbuttered popcorn or berries); or you may need to make a "No Snacks at All" policy for yourself.

For those who can easily stop with one snack serving, your best bet is to keep light and healthful snacks on hand. In my refrigerator, I always keep a bowl of grapes, berries or pre-sliced carrot sticks right on an eye-level shelf. When my family members or I want a snack, the healthful finger foods are right there. I pay a little extra for pre-sliced carrot and celery sticks because I know that if I buy whole carrots, I probably won't get around to slicing them for snacks.

As with the meal guidelines, keep your snacks to one serving between each meal. Here are some suggestions for snacks and recommended serving sizes:

☆ Two cups popcorn, prepared without oil or butter, lightly seasoned with herbs (such as Mrs. Dash) or butter-flavoured sprinkles (such as Butter Buds)

☆ One slice whole-wheat toast, topped with one tablespoon all-fruit spread

☆ One hard-boiled egg

☆ One of the following fruits: a medium apple, a medium banana, one-half medium cantaloupe, a cup of cherries, a medium grapefruit, one-half papaya, a pear, a large peach, a seven-ounce slice of pineapple, two cups of strawberries, two tangerines, or an eleven-ounce slice of watermelon

- ☆ One serving of non-fat yogurt
- ☆ One-quarter cup raisins
- ☆ Two cups carrot sticks
- ☆ Two celery stalks, each spread with reduced-calorie cream cheese
- ☆ Ten whole-wheat, low-salt crackers, plain; or six whole-wheat, low-salt crackers spread with reduced-calorie cream cheese
- ☆ One serving reduced-sodium soup
- ☆ One fat-free corn tortilla, heated in oven until crisp (don't use oil!), then broken into "taco chips" and served with salsa
- ☆ One cup unsweetened apple sauce, sprinkled with cinnamon
- ☆ One honey- or fruit-sweetened cereal bar.

Satisfying Beverages

Water. How many of you have heard the old diet adage to drink eight glasses of water a day, and to drink water right before a meal? If you're like I used to be, you've heard this advice, considered it, and then never quite put it into practice. So when I write that an important part of the Yo-Yo Diet Syndrome plan is to drink those eight glasses of H_2O every day, I know you may ignore me. Yet consider the following facts:

Water is the best defence you have against water retention, bloating and water weight gain. When your diet has too much sodium and salt in it, you may retain water and feel bloated and heavy. A good way to flush out the salt and retained water is by drinking plenty of water.

Water also helps improve the appearance of your skin. Sometimes dieters get what's known as "dieter's pall", meaning a gaunt, haggard look to their faces. Drinking plenty of water is the best way to combat this. Top models know that water is one of the best beauty secrets for looking and feeling great.

Water is also energizing. The next time you feel lethargic or are having an energy slump, reach for a glass of ice water instead of a cup of coffee, and see if you don't feel your energy level pick up. I've found that the colder the water, the more energizing the effect of drinking it is. This energizing effect will help keep you away from snacks during those times when you're apt to reach for a candy bar as an energy booster.

If possible, try to make your water a special beverage by drinking out of a beautifully cut glass or crystal goblet garnished with a slice of lemon or lime. This will help suppress the sense of deprivation that thinking that "it's just a glass of water" brings about. If you don't have ready access to fresh water at work, then bring in your own. Whenever I work outside the home, I carry along a gallon of fresh water. When water is easy to access and in plain view, I'm more likely to drink plenty of it.

Juice. Fruit juice is fairly high in calories, so you'll want to limit how much you drink. However, juice is so healthful, refreshing and invigorating (vitamin C boosts your energy) that I highly recommend its consumption. A glass of juice is a wonderful way to beat the 3:00 p.m. slump that many people experience. One caution is to read the juice's ingredient label to ensure that you are drinking 100 per cent juice and not a "juice drink", "nectar" or "juice blend" containing fructose or corn syrup. Keep in mind that just because a juice is labelled "all natural" doesn't mean that it is "all fruit".

Caffeinated Beverages. I've always held the opinion that no food or liquid is "good" or "bad". So the question is: how does a particular food or beverage make you feel? Does it upset your ability to concentrate? Does it create feelings of jittery anxiety? If so, you're smart to delete that substance from your diet.

My meditation practice led me to conclude that it was best to eliminate most stimulants from my diet if I were to achieve the ability to focus my mind and thoughts at will. When I drink or eat a lot of stimulants, my mind races out of control, focusing on (mostly) negative thoughts. Negative thoughts create negative moods and negative experiences. Therefore, to ensure that my moods and experiences are positive, I have to maintain vigilant awareness and control over the contents of my thoughts. Today, my only source of dietary stimulation is one cup of coffee in the morning. I don't ingest any caffeinated teas, colas or chocolates. Do I feel deprived? Not at all! I actually feel relieved, because now my mind obeys me when I tell it to think positively.

Caffeine, as many of us know, can lead to insomnia or fitful sleep. It's important for Yo-Yo Syndrome dieters to get a good night's sleep, because it is during the dream stage of sleep that the brain produces more serotonin. As you recall, serotonin is the neurotransmitter that regulates mood, energy levels and appetite. Interrupted REM sleep cycles lower the serotonin levels in the brain, which in turn leads to carbohydrate cravings.[1]

Now, I'm not *necessarily* recommending that you eliminate stimulating beverages from your life, although by doing so you're sure to experience pleasant benefits. However, you may want to cut back to an amount that will keep you in control of your thoughts and moods. Here is some of the research about stimulating beverages that may also motivate you to curtail your caffeine consumption:

☆ **Colas.** Yo-Yo Syndrome dieters who are sensitive to mood-altering chemicals are susceptible to caffeine addiction or abuse. Many of my clients have histories of being hooked on diet colas containing caffeine and the aspartame (marketed under NutraSweet) sweetener. These two stimulants give an amphetamine-like rush that some claim lowers their appetite for food. Yo-Yo Syndrome dieters who overeat to quell the emotional pain of disliking their jobs may abuse caffeine to push their bodies to work when their spirits aren't willing.

Studies of aspartame's mood-altering effects have yielded mixed results. However, many documented cases abound of patients complaining of dizziness, lethargy, jitteriness or light-headedness after they ate or drank NutraSweet.[2] However, it appears that part of this chemical's appeal is that it triggers brain production of phenylethylamine, the same chemical created during moments of romantic love. Phenylethylamine is also the same "love drug" found in chocolate.[3]

Although Yo-Yo Syndrome dieters drink diet colas to enjoy a sweet beverage without calories, the ingestion of artificial sweeteners may backfire for well-intentioned dieters. Several studies have concluded that artificial sweeteners *stimulate* the appetite and actually trigger eating binges.[4]

Colas, both diet and regular, deplete your body's magnesium levels, which can drain energy and create food cravings. The phosphoric acid in cola binds with, and extracts, magnesium from the body. Each 12-ounce can of cola removes 36 milligrams of magnesium from the cola drinker's body, according to researcher Kenneth Weaver, MD, of East Tennessee University.

Of course, some non-cola soda-pop flavours also contain caffeine and artificial flavourings and sweeteners. If you're concerned about your caffeine intake, it's a good idea to read the ingredients on that soda-pop can or bottle before you tip it into your mouth.

☆ **Coffee**. Some Yo-Yo Syndrome dieters consume sweetened, flavoured and creamed coffee drinks to curtail cravings for ice cream and other sweets. Artfully prepared coffee drinks are often delicious, even attractive, concoctions. Their popularity is attested to by the swelling ranks of coffee shops anchoring more and more street corners. However, as with cola, I don't believe that coffee is any bargain for dieters. Caffeine and sweeteners stimulate the appetite for food. In the long run, you end up ingesting *more* fat and calories because of the anxiety produced by an overconsumption of caffeine. As a therapist, I have seen neurosis-like anxiety that I believe was triggered by drinking too much coffee.

The appeal of coffee also comes from its tantalizing aroma, which actually contains the mood-altering chemical, pyrazine, which activates the pleasure centre in the brain. That's why the smell of coffee is so pleasant—you're whiffing the brain's "fun chemicals", the same chemicals you experience during silly, playful moments. If your life has been all-work-and-no-play lately, your cravings for coffee probably stem from two factors: first, trying to push yourself to work at a task that you don't want to do; and second, a desire to experience more fun in your life.

If you don't plan on cutting out or down on coffee, you can safeguard your weight-loss programme by:

- ☆ Substituting decaffeinated coffee for regular coffee or blending the two together
- ☆ Avoiding sweeteners, especially artificial ones, which tend to stimulate the appetite for sweet foods
- ☆ Trying a coffee-flavoured grain-based substitute, sold at most health-food stores
- ☆ Avoiding non-dairy creamers, which are loaded with processed and artificial ingredients and are often high in saturated fat
- ☆ Limiting your coffee consumption to the morning hours to avoid insomnia brought about by late-afternoon caffeine ingestion
- ☆ Avoiding real chocolate flavouring in your coffee, as this can lead to overly intense stimulation.

☆ **Tea**.We sometimes think of tea as coffee's charming and innocuous cousin. But it may surprise some people to discover that the innocent-looking cup of tea contains almost as much, if not more, caffeine than a cup of coffee! So if tea is, well, your cup of tea, you'll want to be watchful of caffeine overconsumption. Don't let the dainty china cup handles lull you into a false sense of tranquillity about the ingredients within tea.

Herbal teas are a wonderful beverage alternative for Yo-Yo Syndrome dieters. Some of the more flavourful varieties are available at health-food stores. I personally find the herbal teas produced by the huge commercial tea companies lacking in flavour and freshness. Have fun experimenting with carob tea, orange spice, lemon, apple cinnamon, and camomile (a wonderfully calming and delicately flavoured herb).

You've probably seen, and may have even tried, the so-called dieter's tea. All I can say is, use caution! Many of these teas are supposed to help you lose weight because they contain stimulating herbs, such as mah huang. As with caffeine, even "natural" stimulants can trigger anxiety-based food cravings and binges.

I also believe that any time we become dependent upon a product, even a herb, our self-esteem suffers. If you know, deep down, that you are abusing a chemical such as caffeine, mah huang, melatonin or even camomile, you probably don't feel too good about it. For that reason, it's healthy to use such substances in moderation and to be brutally honest with ourselves about our true motivations for ingesting it.

☆ **Alcohol**. Over the years, I've changed my opinion about whether Yo-Yo Syndrome dieters can mix alcohol into a successful weight-loss and maintenance programme. On the surface, the answer is "of course". After all, a little alcohol in moderation is low in calories and fat. However, from a spiritual-psychological perspective, I recommend abstinence from alcohol, at least during the time when you are attempting to lose weight.

Here's why. The mood-altering effects of alcohol carry over long after the alcohol is emptied from the bloodstream. Alcohol disrupts REM sleep cycles, thus producing a serotonin deficit upon awakening. It's one of the reasons you feel hungover, and it also leads to carbohydrate cravings. The topsy-turvy energy cycles brought on by drinking alcohol also lead to caffeine abuse during the day. As a therapist, I must mention that alcohol can negatively influence one's judgement when interacting with other people. For example, you may have an alcohol-induced argument with your honey. The next day, your mood is doubly dour because of the hangover effect PLUS the fact that you and your lover aren't speaking to one another. You are very likely, at that point, to pour your heart out into a carton of double-chocolate ice cream.

Alcohol also completely interferes with our ability to regulate our thoughts. During normal lucid consciousness, we can easily identify that we are holding a negative thought. Then, we can choose to replace that negative thought with a positive one. In this way, we have a quick reflex in adjusting our moods. This is not the case when we're under the influence, however. Our thoughts become noisy jumbles of negativity, and we can feel helplessly propelled along a torrential stream of downer emotions. It's also very difficult to meditate with a hangover because your concentration goes all over the map. Along the same lines, alcohol can induce us to say, "To heck with my diet!" and eat with total abandon.

From a spiritual standpoint, alcohol weakens and punches holes in the aura in the same way that fluorocarbons puncture the ozone. When this happens, your psychic and healing powers may become limited or inconsistent. Alcohol abuse also attracts earthbound spirits who are often up to no good and who can also rob you of your highest energy levels. These spirits abused alcohol while they were in physical bodies, and they are always looking for vicarious highs from humans. They latch on to their "hosts", so the human then has a spirit jokester or wet-blanket type hanging around. And yes, these spirit personalities do influence our own moods as much as when we are around someone who inhabits a physical body. The best way to uninvite these "guests" is by practising abstinence and avoiding bars and other alcohol- and drug-ridden venues. If you do go to a bar, surround yourself with white light, and say a prayer or archangel invocation before and afterward.[5]

As your intuitive awareness increases, your desires for alcohol and alcohol-related activities will naturally diminish. You simply won't be interested in any activity that takes you away from the excitement inherent in working on your life purpose.

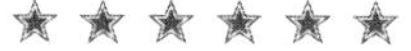

CHAPTER TEN

EXERCISE FOR THE BODY, MIND AND SOUL

"To reach the port of heaven, we must sail sometimes with the wind and sometimes against it, but we must sail, and not drift, nor lie at anchor."

— Oliver Wendell Holmes (1809–1894), physician/author

Throughout time, diet clubs, books and dieting gurus have perpetuated myths and fantasies surrounding weight loss. One myth that unfortunately remains is that you can eat "fat-burning foods" that will give you a trim, toned body without exercising.

I, like many dieters, fought the notion of mandatory exercise for a long time. I thought that I could beat the odds and be different—maybe other people needed to exercise, I rationalized, but not me. So I'd lose weight by vigorous dieting until my body was fairly slim. The trouble was, though, that my diet-thin body was flabby, especially in my stomach, hips and thighs.

Dieting without exercise won't deliver toned muscles or a vibrant energy level. A dramatic example of this was seen in my patient, Chris, a woman who stood 5′4″ tall and weighed 90 pounds. She was, as you may have guessed, suffering from anorexia nervosa. Chris had starved herself from her highest weight of 130 pounds to her present life-threatening weight. Because she refused to eat enough to sustain herself, Chris had to be hospitalized and fed intravenously.

While Chris was in the hospital, the staff took photographs of her while she was standing and clothed in her bra and panties. The purpose was to show Chris how she resembled a skeleton more than a slim fashion model. When she saw the photos of herself, Chris was shocked!

"I couldn't believe what I looked like!" she told me. "My hips and thighs were completely out of proportion with the rest of my body." It was true. Chris had believed she'd get the body of a high-fashion model if only she'd starve herself to a certain thinness. She never exercised, however—mostly because her starving made her too weak to do anything physical. But the striking thing for Chris to realize was that, without exercise, she'd never have the firm stomach and thighs that she dreamed of. Chris had starved herself into a cartoon-like, distorted version of her former self.

Of course, anorexia nervosa is an extreme example of someone who is starving for love. Chris believed that if she had a perfect body, her husband would love her more (and Chris thought that she would love herself more if this happened). So her therapy was focused on psychological and spiritual treatments of her seeming love deficit. However, Chris's case definitely highlights how we can't starve our way to a healthy body or a healthy self-image. We only become flabby, skinny people without exercise.

There are several other important benefits you'll get from exercise:

☆ Your weight loss will be faster.

☆ Your appetite will lessen, along with your cravings for binge foods and snacks.

☆ Your brain's serotonin level will be boosted from aerobic-type exercise, which stabilizes your mood, energy and appetite.[1]

☆ You will feel more energetic during the day.[1]

☆ You will sleep more soundly and wake up more refreshed.[2]

☆ You will find that your stress level is reduced (great news for Stress Eaters!).[2]

☆ You will find that your fattening feelings are reduced (great news for Emotion Eaters!). [3]

The exercise programme described below is designed with the sedentary, unmotivated person in mind. Of course, it's wise to consult your primary physician before embarking on an exercise programme. This particular exercise programme *gradually* introduces you to a regular fitness routine.

Develop and Choose Your Exercise Programme

The consensus among fitness experts is that aerobic-type activity—the kind that gets your heart pumping, your rate of breathing up and your pores perspiring—is the best way to lose fat and improve your cardiovascular fitness. Getting your heart rate up to target level for at least 40 minutes at a time is generally considered better for your weight-loss programme than exercising less strenuously for longer periods of time. That's why normal housework isn't a viable substitute for aerobic activity. (To calculate your target heart rate, refer back to the box on page 126.)

Ideally, you will choose aerobic-type activities, such as those described below, and perform them at your target heart rate for at least 40 continuous minutes four or more times a week. However, I realize that this isn't palatable or feasible for every reader, so there are alternative suggestions following this section. The important point is to get in the habit of moving your body, and enjoying the activity as well.

When exercising, avoid exceeding your target heart rate, as this will put you into the anaerobic process, in which you're building muscle instead of burning fat. Always warm up slowly for at least five minutes before exercising aerobically, and cool down after exercising until your heart rate is at least 15 beats per minute below your target heart rate.

It's also important to drink plenty of water after, or even during, exercise to avoid dehydration. And at the risk of sounding like a nagging physical-education teacher, let me also strongly suggest that you invest in a good pair of sturdy athletic shoes that are made for your particular sport. Any sporting goods store can give you a mini-education about the athletic-shoe varieties if you need more information.

Low-Impact Aerobics. This form of aerobics is different from that of the '70s and '80s, where people bounced and swung their bodies in sometimes injurious ways. Low-impact aerobic classes are offered at most gyms, on television programmes and on DVDs or videos. I would try out the classes before signing a long-term agreement with the gym, to ensure that you feel comfortable with the instructors, the room temperature and the class schedule. There are also many specialized aerobics classes, such as those for plus-size women and for expectant mothers. Variations on low-impact aerobics include "step classes", where participants step up and down on a single stair step; and "rubber-band classes", which combine aerobics with a lightweight workout achieved by stretching a rubber band.

Jogging. This is a nice exercise to engage in before or after work, and it can be made even more enjoyable by listening to an inspiring CD or radio programme. You may choose to jog around your neighbourhood, on a track at a nearby school or college, or on a scenic path near a lake or park. If you haven't jogged much, you may want to read about safety considerations and techniques in jogging books available at your local library or sporting-goods store.

Rebounder (Trampoline) Jogging. This relatively inexpensive piece of exercise equipment is available at most department and sporting-goods stores, and is ideal for people who prefer to exercise at home. There are books and tapes that describe different ways to exercise on the rebounder. In addition, many people bounce while holding five- to ten-pound weights or strapping weights on their wrists or ankles to increase the amount of calories they burn.

Swimming. You can burn calories and tone muscles by swimming laps back and forth across the pool or by doing calisthenics, letting the resistance of the water pump up your heart and calorie-burning rate. Some studies show that the rate of calorie burning is not as intense in a cold swimming pool as it is in non-water sports, because the body conserves calories when it is cold.

Stair Climbing. This is my personal favourite. I use a StairMaster machine, which simulates walking, jogging or running up flights of stairs. Stair climbing is superb for toning the buttocks and legs, as well as burning calories and building cardiovascular fitness. I also like stair machines because it is easy to read during exercise, which keeps me from getting bored and helps me catch up on my reading.

Most gyms have stair-climbing machines. However, if yours doesn't, or if you don't go to a gym, you can still get the benefit of stair climbing by stepping up and down on a small, sturdy box. Or you can imitate professional athletes by running up and down the grandstand steps at your local football field.

Bicycle Riding. If you don't own a bicycle, either stationary or conventional, think about investing in one. There's nothing more relaxing than pedalling to the local grocery store or just tooling around the neighbourhood at sunset. Bicycling is also ideal for involving your family in your exercise programme.

Stationary bicycles are handy for at-home fitness buffs, as you can park them in front of the television set and pedal away as you watch your favourite show. Many gyms offer "spinning" classes, similar to aerobics classes, except group members and the instructor are all on stationary bicycles. In addition, sporting-goods stores offer DVDs or videos made especially for stationary bicycle riding.

These DVDs simulate how it would feel to ride your bicycle on windy mountain roads and other picturesque trails. I'm also impressed with recumbent stationary bicycles, which allow you to recline while pedalling—a very comfortable way to work out, indeed! Since so many different manufacturers produce a similar type of machine, I would test any product before purchasing it to ensure that it feels comfortable and sturdy.

Stationary Ski Machines. My clients and friends who have these machines (usually thought of as a NordicTrack, but also manufactured by other companies) seem to fall into two categories: those who love it and report great results, and those who find the machine awkward to use and who end up stowing it permanently underneath their beds. If you love a challenging and intense workout, you just may find that a stationary ski machine fits the bill for you.

Rowing. Rowing machines are another piece of equipment that you can add to your home fitness centre or use at the local gym. If you live near a body of water, why not row a real boat or kayak for a great workout with plenty of fresh air? Rowing is great for building up a sweat and getting an aerobic workout, and it tones the arms, chest and shoulders as well. Many electronic rowing machines add visual interest and excitement to the workout by simulating a video game where you are racing another rowing boat.

Rollerskating and Inline Skating. Remember when you were little and you'd strap on your skates for a whirl around the block? As you may know, our childhood sport is now all grown up. I was avidly into inline skating until I took a few spills that turned me off this sport. But many people enjoy the speed and freedom of skating across the cement. Skating is a great workout, and it tones the inner and outer thighs, as well as the buttocks. I definitely recommend taking classes if you want to try inline skating, and please don't forget that safety pads and helmets are a must.

★ ★ ★

Tennis. I like tennis because it's a social sport, and exercising with a friend can help keep Yo-Yo Syndrome dieters motivated to stick with their fitness programmes. You and your tennis partner can make sure you both get out on the court—no excuses accepted.

Brisk Walking/Treadmills. I have a fold-up treadmill that saves space when it's not in use. On rainy days, or late at night when I don't care to exercise outdoors, I love using my treadmill. It's also ideal for exercising while listening to a CD programme. Brisk walking is another exercise that's best done with a partner, either human or canine. This exercise is a good way to combine soulful conversations with a workout (more walking information follows).

Rock Climbing, Backpacking and Hiking. If you love the great outdoors and you're the adventurous sort, what could be better than packing some supplies and heading out into a nature area with a friend or family member? Many sporting-goods stores offer rock-climbing classes, which provide a great social outlet for meeting new friends or romantic interests.

Those are brief explanations of just a few of the many aerobic-type exercises you could choose from. You can get additional workout ideas and inspiration by reading fitness magazines such as *Shape*, *Zest*, *Men's Health* or *Women's Health*. Your local gym may offer workout classes that are fun, new and innovative. Check their class schedules to see what appeals to you.

I also recommend looking for used or consignment sporting-goods stores that offer workout equipment for a fraction of the new cost. You can find them in the yellow pages under "Sports Equipment, Used" or "Sporting Goods, Used". Look for any equipment warranties or guarantees that may be transferable or that the store offers.

Walking: Setting You Off in the Right Direction

I realize that not everyone is going to gleefully jump into a fitness programme. Many regard exercising as a chore and painfully recall gruelling high-school physical-education classes when they had to run ten laps around the schoolyard. Some will say, "Well, I'll try the rest of this book's suggestions, but I'll skip the exercise part." Others, who have been sedentary for six months or more, are wise to avoid diving into an aerobics-type programme. Instead, they need to gradually incorporate exercise into their lifestyles.

Walking is a pain-free way to gently introduce exercise into your life and help you burn fat and calories. Although this is not an aerobic programme (unless you walk briskly), it will start you in the right direction and perhaps inspire you to move on to an aerobics programme later.

The walking programme involves adding three activities to your normal daily routine:

1. If you drive or ride in a car, always park your auto at the outer edge of the parking lot. If you take public transportation, and it is safe and feasible, leave the train or bus one exit before your normal getting-off point. This will give you opportunities to walk to your destination, and it will also save your car from "parking-lot dings".

2. Take the stairs instead of the lift or escalator. You'll beat the crowds and will probably get to your destination faster than you would by waiting around for the lift to arrive.

3. Once a day, go for a half-hour walk around the neighbourhood or the area in which you work. Make this a firm rule for yourself, and always stick to it. After-dinner overeaters are wise to adopt the habit of getting out of the kitchen, out of the house, and outside into the fresh air. Homemakers, shift workers and those who work out of their homes could take morning walks to get their metabolism going and inspire them to avoid overeating during the day. Others could take their walking shoes to work and take a brisk walk during lunchtime. This is a natural way to burn calories and avoid the temptation to overeat during lunch.

Exercise, once incorporated into your lifestyle, has a ripple effect that creates an all-around healthy mindset. After going to the time and trouble to exercise, you're not as apt to spoil your efforts with overeating.

If your schedule doesn't permit a walk because you get home so late at night (or if you don't feel safe walking around your neighbourhood), go for a walk at the local shopping centre or mall. Just be sure to stay away from the dessert shops! Or you could walk in place or use a treadmill on slow speed while watching your favourite television show.

What Kind of Exercise Do You Prefer?

Please don't make the mistake of waiting until you're in the mood to begin an exercise programme, because that day may never come. Instead, push yourself to do something physical right now.

If you don't belong to a gym, then maybe it's time to join one. Exercising at home alone requires a tremendous amount of self-discipline—something most of us don't have when we're first starting a diet and fitness programme. Pick a gym where you feel comfortable, which is located close enough to your home or workplace so that you'll actually go there at least four times a week.

Many Yo-Yo Syndrome dieters are embarrassed to join a gym, thinking that they're too overweight to exercise in shorts in front of strangers. I understand this illogical logic, because I've thought the same thing in years past. It's kind of like wanting to clean your home before the housekeeper arrives so she won't think you're a slob. However, don't fall into this trap now, because gyms are there to help you tone your muscles and lose your excess weight. Besides, I've found that most people working out at gyms—male and female—are too absorbed in their own worlds to notice those exercising around them.

It's really important that you choose an activity that you enjoy, or it will be even more difficult to talk yourself into exercising. Think about your natural tendencies when deciding what type of exercise to engage in:

- ☆ Do you prefer to be alone? Then you'll probably do best exercising at home. Since you won't have anyone around urging you to exercise, you'll have to schedule exercise into your lifestyle. You may want to do this by pairing another activity that is already an ingrained habit—say, your two o'clock soap opera or your four o'clock talk radio show—with the exercise. This will trigger a reminder that it's time to watch "Days of Our Lives" or listen to your call-in show *and* jog on the rebounder.
- ☆ Do you prefer to be with one other person? Then you may enjoy two-person sports such as tennis or racquet-

ball. This may be an ideal situation as well, if you and your exercise buddy make a pact to gently "bully" each other into working out on those days when you'd rather not.

- ☆ Do you like to be with a *lot* of other people? If so, then you'll probably like gyms, aerobics, yoga, martial arts or dance classes. At these places, you'll have the opportunity to introduce yourself to new friends.

- ☆ Do you like to be indoors? Then choose exercises that take place in gyms, tennis courts, martial arts studios, dance halls or indoor swimming pools—or exercise at home.

- ☆ Do you prefer the outdoors? Then your sports would naturally be in league with tennis, bicycle riding, team sports, kayaking, jogging, hiking or brisk walking.

- ☆ Do you want to lower your stress level? Then you'd be happiest with a mind–body–spirit fitness programme such as yoga, tai chi or rock climbing.

- ☆ Do you want to tone your muscles? Your ideal sport will involve weight workouts, such as free weights, weight equipment, yoga, jogging on sandy soil, or rubber band classes.

There are other considerations to keep in mind—for example, your budget. Some exercise programmes, such as tennis or gym memberships, can run into a great deal of money by the time you finish paying for gym outfits, workout shoes and club dues. When I belonged to a gym, I was primarily using the stair climber and free weights. I found that it was less expensive to purchase my own stair climber and free weights, and save the cost of the monthly club dues (plus avoid the lines that invariably formed to use the stair climber). Other workout programmes, such as brisk walking or using an exercise video, cost practically nothing (although you should make sure to wear proper shoes no matter what exercise you choose).

Keep Yourself Motivated

How many times have you joined a gym, bought some home-exercise equipment, or committed yourself to a jogging regime, only to abandon it a month later? If you're like most Yo-Yo Syndrome dieters, the answer's likely to be, "Too many times to remember."

Exercise, while such an important part of any weight-loss programme, is usually the first thing to fall by the wayside when schedules get busy. For some, getting started is the hardest part, but then once these people get into a routine of exercising, they begin to enjoy it so much that they refuse to let it go. But for most of us, sticking with exercise is the hard part. We'll run, pump or swim ourselves into shape and then stop exercising for one reason or another. And when we stop working out, we often return to overeating. This time, plan on sticking with your fitness routine!

Remember, there are no stopping points for exercising. We don't just get in shape one day and say, "Okay, that's enough exercise. I'm done with it forever."

Here are some tips that will help you to stick with your exercise programme. Try them out—they really do help!

- ☆ If you like the sport you've chosen, you're more likely to stick with it. Keep in mind that it may take time to find the activity that's right for you, so be patient if the one you're currently engaged in doesn't feel quite right. Instead of abandoning exercise entirely, switch to a different type.

- ☆ Schedule exercise into your day in the same way you would any important activity. Plan ahead which days and times would be best for you to exercise; note in pen on your calendar which days you plan to exercise. Try to be realistic in scheduling your exercise time to avoid setting yourself up for frustration. Also, plan your exercise around your peak energy time (for example, if you're a "morning person", plan to exercise in the a.m. hours), and you'll feel more like working out.

- ☆ Don't look at exercise as optional. Just as you wouldn't dream of missing that important meeting or doctor's appointment, keep your promise to yourself and exercise every time it's written on your calendar.

- ☆ If you begin to argue with yourself about why you don't have time to exercise, *stop*! Don't give yourself time to even consider not exercising. You don't stop and argue with yourself about whether to shower every day, do you? Of course not! Do you stop and say, "Well, I don't have time to brush my hair and my teeth"? No. Put exercise into this category of things you naturally do, such as dressing and grooming yourself.

- ☆ Buy a new exercise outfit or some new workout shoes. There's nothing like feeling attractive to give you the incentive to exercise. Just as you feel more excited about going to work when dressed in a flattering new outfit, you'll feel more charged-up about exercising if you know that you look your best.

- ☆ Reward yourself for exercising, but wait until after your workout to do so. For instance, you can withhold your evening snack until after you're done working out. Or put a pound into a piggy bank every time you exercise, and spend it on yourself once a week or once a month.

- ☆ Pray for spiritual assistance in establishing your motivation to take good care of your body. God provides for *all* our needs, including our emotional ones. However, we must remember to ask for help.

- ☆ Team sports can add fun to your exercise programme as well as keep you motivated (there's nothing like a play-off schedule to force you to exercise). Call your local parks and recreation department or community college and ask about joining their netball, football or softball team.

- ☆ Consider hiring a personal trainer. This person will help you construct a fitness routine to suit your goals and needs. Then the trainer will accompany you during your entire workout—either at home or the gym—to make sure you complete each exercise safely and thoroughly. A smart friend of mine *prepaid* her personal trainer for three months of workouts. In that way, she ensured that she wouldn't quit exercising as she'd done so many times in the past. Plus, she received a great cost reduction for prepaying. To find out the cost of a trainer (some even work on the barter system—just ask them), call your local gyms.

- ☆ Exercising with a friend is another way to keep your motivation high, have fun and have someone to talk to while you work out. Make a pact with one another not to accept any excuses for not exercising, and you'll be able to push each other into sticking with a fitness routine.

☆ Form a walking club with your neighbours. Four or five of you walking together will provide lots of stimulating conversation, and you may feel safer walking in a group.

☆ Like dieting, take your exercise programme one day at a time. Set small goals for yourself, and be patient as you gradually increase your running distance, build aerobic stamina or lift progressively more weight. Try not to compare yourself to others, except as a way to set future goals for yourself.

☆ No excuses (except illness or injury) are acceptable for missing your exercise routine. If, after being brutally honest with yourself about your reasons, you decide you really can't exercise this morning as you planned, then reschedule your workout for this evening. Remember, excuses won't get the weight off.

☆ Some people drop out of exercise programmes because they've overdone it and have experienced "exercise burn-out". Be realistic when scheduling exercise into your life, and maintain a balance between too little and too much of a workout.

☆ Going away to a hotel for the weekend or for a business conference? Don't let your fitness routine be interrupted. This often breaks the pattern of exercising and may cause you to stop your fitness programme altogether. Make your reservations only at hotels that feature work-out rooms, gyms, information on nearby health clubs with cooperative arrangements for hotel guests, or jogging paths.

- ☆ I, like many of my clients, have found that aerobic-type exercise sparks creative ideas. I believe it has to do with the increased oxygen intake and serotonin production. For that reason, you might want to carry a small tape recorder or paper and pencil as you work out, to capture your ideas as they occur. This benefit will help reinforce the rewards of exercising, especially for Stress Eaters who often claim that their heavy workload prevents them from exercising.

- ☆ Finally, if your motivation to exercise is really low, try my 15-Minute Personal Pact. Tell yourself, "I'll exercise for 15 minutes. If after 15 minutes, I feel like stopping, I will stop. After all, 15 minutes of exercise is better than nothing." I can virtually guarantee you that after 15 minutes, you'll want to keep going and you'll end up exercising for your 40-minute workout.

Exercising regularly is as important as any of the other steps involved in healing the Yo-Yo Diet Syndrome, so please don't skip it. Too many studies confirm that toned, fit bodies are the result of combining a low-calorie, low-fat diet with exercise. Remember: exercise is not optional!

CHAPTER ELEVEN

LIFESTYLE STRATEGIES FOR THE YO-YO DIET SYNDROME

"Excessive eating is prejudicial to health, to fame, and to bliss in Heaven; it prevents the acquisition of spiritual merit and is odious among men; one ought, for these reasons, to avoid it carefully."

— Hinduism, *Laws of Manu* 2.57

Yo-Yo Syndrome dieters often worry about how to avoid overeating while away from home. Due to the myriad pressures and temptations that arise when you go "out there", Yo-Yo Syndrome dieters do need to stay on guard to avoid overeating and subsequent weight gains.

There's no doubt about it—a weight-loss programme often requires tremendous commitment in the face of temptation, stress or strong emotions. There's the dessert cart the waitress pushes under your nose. The birthday cake at work. Aunt Mary's holiday sugar cookies. And the tempting buffets of exotic foods offered on cruise ships, at weddings and parties, and at all-you-can-eat restaurants. Sometimes it feels as if the whole world is ganging up on you, in one huge effort to get you to overeat. What's a Yo-Yo Syndrome dieter to do?

Although I had one client who actually tried to arrange her life so that she never had to eat a meal away from home, most of us can't—or don't want to—avoid eating in restaurants, at friends' homes or at parties. And you don't have to!

This chapter focuses on ways to keep your yo-yoing under control, despite roadblocks and hurdles that invariably arise. Just as you can improve your chances of surviving a fire by planning an escape route ahead of time, you can benefit from learning how to avoid these common overeating traps.

This chapter gives you some tools for survival and some ways to keep your Yo-Yo Diet Syndrome in check. But by far, the greatest tool that you'll carry with you, both in your home and out of it, is the knowledge that you alone are responsible for what goes in your mouth (or on your thighs or belt line). No matter what pressures come up in your life, no matter how guilty you may feel about saying no to someone's cooking, remember that you are in control of everything you eat.

Restaurants—Eating Out and Eating Light

When dining out, you'll need to be very honest with yourself about how much food you're going to eat. Many restaurants are notorious for serving extra-big portions of food; often, the equivalent of two normal servings appears on the large plate set before you. Since healing the Yo-Yo Diet Syndrome entails eating only one serving of whatever you consume, you'll need to stop eating when you start to feel full. You need to remind yourself that a full plate is not the waiter's way of giving you implied permission to overeat! Use your judgment to figure out how much food equals one serving. But, yes, I realize that the temptation to "eat the whole thing" often wins out, so here are some tips that may help:

- ☆ Before ordering, look at the size of the meals being served to the other restaurant patrons. Do they look like normal-, medium- or gigantic-sized portions?

- ☆ If they look gigantic, ask your waiter if you can order a half-meal. Most restaurants are more than happy to accommodate such requests. By having a smaller meal in front of you, you'll be less tempted to overeat.

- ☆ If you feel comfortable with the idea, why not split a gigantic meal with your dining companion? Even if there is a slight extra charge for splitting a meal, it's worth it in calorie savings.

- ☆ Remember that leaving food on your plate isn't wasteful. What *is* wasteful is eating more than you need and being angry at yourself for the extra weight you may subsequently gain.

- ☆ Focus on the conversation among your dining companions, and take your attention away from your meal. Practise the healthful habit of putting your eating utensils down between bites to avoid gobbling.

- ☆ As soon as you begin to feel full (not stuffed), do one of the following before you even have time to think about eating more: throw your napkin over the plate so you won't see the remaining food; take someone's cigarette and put it out in the food; or sprinkle pepper, sugar or Tabasco sauce all over the food on your plate—anything to make it less appealing to you.

Don't even let yourself entertain the notion of eating more if you're full, *regardless* of how delicious the meal tastes to you. Push your plate to the edge of the table to alert the waiter/waitress that you are finished eating and that you want your plate removed. After ten or 15 minutes, your brain should catch up with your stomach and register signals that it's full of food. In the meantime, you can go to the restroom and brush your teeth (be sure to carry a toothbrush and toothpaste with you at all times). Then order sparkling mineral water or juice blended with slushed ice so you don't feel empty-handed if your dining companions are still eating.

Some Words of Advice for Binge Eaters

If you are a Binge Eater, please don't play the game that so many do: you see that the food on your restaurant plate contains your binge food. It looks delicious. You want it. So you tell yourself, "I can pretend I didn't know my binge food was in this meal, and then it really wouldn't be my fault if I ate it." Yes, it may not be your "fault" that you ate the food, but you'll be the one who ends up going on an eating binge. You'll be the one who feels fat, miserable and out of control. That's why it's vital to take responsibility for what you eat.

If you ever confront that dilemma of trying to decide, "Is it okay to eat my binge food or not?" remember that you really don't even have the option. If you eat the binge food, you will end up relapsing—either today or in the next few days. And binges are not to be taken lightly, because they're difficult to stop and damaging to the self-esteem.

Remember: "*If it is to be, it's up to me.*"

Going to a restaurant doesn't mean engaging in a struggle with your binge food. There are plenty of ways to stay on your diet programme and feel very satisfied with your meal. The main thing to keep in mind when you eat out is that even a little taste of your binge food could trigger overeating, so carefully investigate how the meal is prepared before you order it. Don't be shy about asking waiters and waitresses questions about the dish; it's part of their job to give you information about the foods you order. Some possible queries are listed below.

☆ Bread bingers might ask if meat dishes are breaded or if the soup is thickened with flour. Ask that the side of toast, biscuits or bread either not be served, be given to your non-bread-bingeing eating companion, or be replaced by an extra portion of vegetables.

☆ Sugar bingers might inquire whether sugar is included in the meal's ingredients, especially if it's hidden in sauces, vegetables, dressings and salads.

☆ Salty-junk-food bingers need to particularly avoid deep-fried crunchy foods, and therefore they need to ask how meat dishes are prepared.

☆ Spicy-food bingers must ask whether ingredients can be substituted to tone down the intensity of the meal. These days, the better restaurants are accustomed to preparing low-sodium menus, and special requests are welcomed.

☆ Feel free to ask for meals that are not spicy, and you will find that your request is accommodated with grace. If not, maybe you'll reconsider eating in that restaurant, or you could ask for the blander things on the menu.

☆ Dairy-product bingers need to find out if their binge food was used as part of the meal's preparation. If your binge food is cheese, then ask to have the order prepared without it—a very reasonable request that probably won't give the restaurant staff any trouble. Be sure, before you order, that your meal won't be smothered with white sauce. And, of course, order a non-dairy dressing with your dinner salad.

As long as you avoid your binge food, you'll probably be able to eat at any restaurant without feeling that your appetite is out of control.

Tips on Travelling Without Overeating

The guidelines for restaurants are also applicable while you're travelling or on vacation. In fact, it would be a good idea to pack this book in your suitcase for reference while you're away from home. Most people complain about gaining weight while they're on vacation, and there are lots of reasons why this is so.

The first is that a lot of us have unrealistic expectations about how we'll feel before we go on vacation. Consider the couple, for instance, who save for ten years and dream of the day when they can go on a cruise to the Bahamas. The wife fantasizes about feeling elegant as she dines with the captain and dances in her evening gowns, while her husband dreams about lolling about on the deck and taking long snoozes in the afternoon sun.

Since this husband and wife have different mental pictures and expectations—all of which are sure to fall short of reality—they're likely to feel somewhat let down, frustrated and angry while they're on the cruise. After all those years of saving money and dreaming, they may feel cheated when the actual cruise doesn't match their fantasies.

Since cruise ships are notorious for offering round-the-clock buffets, how do you think Mr. and Mrs. Disappointed will spend their time? They will probably stuff their disappointment with all-you-can-eat meals.

In the same vein, the busy executive who dreams all year of the two weeks in July when he can relax in Maui may also be setting himself up for an eating binge. Once he gets to the Hawaiian island, he may feel as keyed up as he does at the office, so he Stress Eats to try to relax. Or he finds that the hordes of tourists are extremely unpleasant, so he tries to unwind and escape by overindulging in food at the restaurants that line the island shores.

Our unmet expectations about vacations can lead to disappointment, anger, anxiety, frustration and depression—all feelings that place us at high risk for Emotion Eating. As a result, it's important to be realistic about your vacation. Try not to look at your trip as a magical cure-all for all your stresses and problems. Basically you will be the same person on your vacation, with the same body and personality. Not that much will change, except for the scenery.

Yes, vacations are wonderful. But they're better when you keep your expectations about them down-to-earth and simple. Dream about being able to get away from phones and work. Look forward to the pretty vistas you'll encounter. And yes, you'll probably be able to relax and have some fun, too. If you keep your fantasies in check, you won't trigger the fattening feelings that lead Emotion Eaters to overeat.

The second major reason why vacations lead to overeating is the fatigue that accompanies travel and erratic schedules. If you travel by plane to another time zone, drive hundreds of miles, sleep in strange quarters, or party all night, your body's going to let you know that it's tired. And, as you may remember from the chapter on Emotion Eaters, being tired—experiencing "fatigue"—is the second most common feeling leading to Emotion Eating. We try to boost our energy by eating, when what we really need is sleep.

For this reason, it's a good idea to plan your vacation so that you're able to rest and relax as much as possible. Plan your arrival so that you can nap for an hour or two after checking in to the hotel. Don't expect to drive more hours than your body can withstand. Try to stay in hotels with comfortable accommodations, and ask for a quiet room away from noisy traffic areas including vending machines and lifts. Of course, don't abuse your body by staying up all night or overindulging in alcohol. Taking these measures will help you withstand the temptation to Emotion Eat or Stress Eat.

Another factor involved in vacation-time overeating is having more time and more opportunity than normal to eat. Someone who's not used to relaxing, for instance, may feel uncomfortable with all the unstructured vacation time and try to fill those hours with food-related activities. For example, they may spend their time reading about the local restaurants, planning where to go for dinner that evening, calling to make reservations for upcoming meals, driving to the restaurant, and then, of course, eating. This alone can use up hours in a day.

As I touched on before, people who go on cruises get even more opportunities to overeat, because most cruises serve all-you-can-eat buffets several times a day. Those Yo-Yo Syndrome dieters who worry about getting their money's worth, or who feel anxious about missing something, may fall into the trap of bingeing their way through the Caribbean.

In addition, many Snowball Effect Eaters overindulge on vacation because they confuse eating with entertainment. They think of gorging on food as part of the fun of travelling, so they end up overeating in this misguided "recreation". However, instead of feeling elated, they feel fat. Finally, vacations often end in enormous weight additions because Binge Eaters eat their binge foods.

Your vacation probably comes just once a year, maybe even less often. It is meant to be a happy, memorable time in your life. By staying on your diet plan during your travels, you'll feel better physically and emotionally.

Here are some tips, then, to keep in mind during your travels:

☆ Maintain your exercise programme while you're on vacation. While you may not have access to the same type of exercise equipment or setting you have at home, be sure to engage in some sort of physical activity each day. Try something new and fun such as dancing, swimming, snorkelling, tennis, kayaking or racquetball. The benefits include:

- ☆ Keeping your muscles toned
- ☆ Burning fat and calories
- ☆ Reducing fattening feelings and stress
- ☆ Giving you healthy, non-food fun and entertainment
- ☆ Helping maintain your motivation for dieting
- ☆ Allowing you to keep your energy level higher
- ☆ Providing structured time, thereby reducing the chances that you'll eat out of boredom.

☆ Continue to plan your meals ahead of time. You can do so, even when you're on vacation, by reading the menu of the restaurant you plan to go to (usually found in hotel publications, travel guide magazines and on display in front of the restaurant) *before* you get inside the restaurant. Decide on a meal that fits your diet plan before you sit down at the restaurant table so that impulsiveness or "the eyes bigger than the stomach" syndrome doesn't trigger overeating.

If you're eating at a buffet, then use the guidelines given in Chapter Nine: walk around the entire buffet first, and note what looks good to you and what foods fit your diet plan. Then choose up to six items that will fulfil your quota for foods from the dairy, starch, meat and fruit/vegetable groups for that meal. And remember to eat one serving only!

☆ Sightseers and vacationers travelling by car must be especially alert to stay on their diets. In an effort to conserve time and money, many motorists cut corners at mealtime, and this can be disastrous for a diet! The following tips will help keep you on track:

First, if most of your meals are eaten at fast-food restaurants, try to stick to salads to avoid overdoing fatty fried foods and red meats. Second, don't keep snacks in the car, as the distractions of driving make many people overeat without realizing it. Instead, eat your snacks right after lunch and dinner so that they're more controlled. Finally, get out of the car for fresh air, and exercise at least twice a day to keep your energy level up and reduce "fat-igue".

☆ Airplane travellers can reduce their chances of overeating by taking two important steps. First, because food served on airlines is often greasy, salty and difficult to digest during air travel, it's best to call the airline ahead of time and request a vegetarian meal or some healthful fare (something that most airlines provide for every passenger who asks). A special meal will contain fewer calories and less sodium and fat, which will make you feel more refreshed when you arrive at your destination.

Second, plan your meals according to your destination's time zone. When travelling to a different part of the world, it's easy to get mixed up about whether it's time for breakfast, lunch or dinner. On one trip I took many years ago—when my weight was still yo-yoing—I ate breakfast before driving to the airport for my 10:00 a.m. flight to Hawaii (which is three hours behind my state's time zone). When I was on the flight, the staff served breakfast, which I ate. Then, when I arrived at my hotel in Hawaii, it was one o'clock (island time), so I ate lunch. My body, tired from the flight and still accustomed to California time, felt as if it was approaching dinnertime (4:00 p.m.). This meant I ate a larger-than-normal lunch. And that evening, I had a big dinner. Eating four large meals that first day of my vacation set me up to continue a food-centred holiday for my entire Hawaiian stay, and I gained ten pounds in 11 days. To combat this now, I plan my eating schedule ahead of time. If I'm taking a breakfast flight, I don't eat before going to the airport. I plan according to the time zone I'm travelling to so I know when and where I'll be eating each meal. In this way, I reduce confusion about meal times and stick with my three daily meals.

☆ Plan your vacation itinerary around activities not involving food. Instead of making your restaurant trips the highlight of the day, plan your day around a journey to a famous landmark. Or play a game with yourself or your companions about how much money you can save by eating light. Then, spend the extra money on a special non-food treat for yourself (such as a new outfit, theatre tickets or a helicopter ride). You'll remember these things a lot longer than you would a heavy meal.

☆ Stress Eaters and Emotion Eaters: you must be sure to get enough relaxation and rest during your vacations. It's important to slow down from your normal hectic pace while you're on holiday. Guard against the habit of filling up each moment with activity, and allow for some lazing about and spontaneity during each day. Keep up your daily meditation routines in order to stay connected to the serenity of your spirit and soul.

Your Food-Filled Holiday and Birthday Survival Guide

Many Yo-Yo Syndrome dieters have childhood memories of Christmases spent eating delicious cookies, and Passovers where eating huge amounts of food was the main attraction. Holidays and food just seem to go hand-in-hand for most of us, making these times of the year very precarious when it comes to our weight.

The emotional roller coaster that accompanies holidays can make this an especially difficult time of year for Emotion Eaters. There are feelings of loneliness connected to being away from your family at Christmas, grief resulting from loved ones who are no longer with you, sadness that you're no longer a child on Easter morning, and disappointment that your birthday wasn't remembered. Conversely, feelings of happiness and a desire to celebrate can also lead to food cravings for Emotion Eaters.

Holidays can be like vacations in that they are filled with unrealistic expectations that can lead to emotional overeating. We may dream about the gifts we'll get for our birthday, and we may unconsciously expect holidays to be similar to the happier ones we experienced as children. All these expectations set Emotion Eaters up for fattening feelings such as disappointment and emptiness.

For many of us, holidays mean going home again, and there's a particular tendency to want to eat when you go to your parents' home. A friend of mine who's a Yo-Yo Syndrome dieter told me that the minute she sets foot in her parents' home (the same one she grew up in), she makes a beeline for the refrigerator. Thinking about her reasons for doing this, she discovered that going home makes her feel like a little girl again. And, as a little girl, she used to overeat a great deal. In other words, she has correlated being home with eating Mum's cooking.

Ruth, a client of mine, tells me that her mother keeps candy in the same kitchen drawer today that she did when Ruth was a young girl. Every time Ruth goes home to visit her mother, she can barely keep from opening "the candy drawer" because it's such a powerful habit.

Still another client, Liz, tells me that when she goes home for the holidays, her mother frets over her by continually saying,

"Liz, you're much too thin!" Then Liz's mother insists that she eat something, which Liz is more than happy to do since she loves her mother's baking.

The guidelines for eating during the holidays are the same as during any other day of the year. Your body, after all, never takes a day off from turning excess calories into body fat. Therefore, there's no special occasion to warrant overeating—even if Aunt Martha has prepared something just for you!

Snowball Effect Eaters and Emotion Eaters pair food with celebration, so they see holidays and birthdays as a logical excuse to overeat. Not overeating on a special occasion is tantamount to deprivation, according to Snowball Effect Eaters. That's why it's so important to recognize and break this mindset. Otherwise, Snowball Effect Eaters will overeat at every conceivable celebratory occasion—and there are a lot of holidays, celebrations and birthdays packed into each year.

But in some households, I realize that there is a pressure to overeat at family occasions. You may feel you're hurting Grandma's feelings if you turn down some of her cooking, even if it is your binge food. What can you do in cases like this? Well, you could use the tactic well-known to all children: put a single serving on your plate, and then push it around with your fork so that it looks as if you've eaten some.

I believe the best approach, though, is to spend most of your holiday time talking and listening to your family members, and spend less time eating food. That way, your plate will stay full with your first course during the time when your cousins, sisters, aunts and uncles are dishing up their third helpings. Eat slowly, put your fork down between bites, and drink plenty of water. If someone asks you if you want more food, simply but firmly state, "I'm so full!" How can anyone argue with you if you announce that you are satiated?

If, on the other hand, you tell your family that you are "on a diet", beware! You're likely to get an earful of dieting advice and admonitions of "Why are you on a diet? You're not fat!" While we all like to get compliments, sometimes these well-meaning statements give us implied permission to go on an eating binge. After all, if Uncle Mark says we're not fat, it must be so!

More Holiday Advice

Since Yo-Yo Syndrome dieters often have an especially difficult time at Halloween, Easter, Passover, Hanukkah and Christmas, when candy and desserts are so prevalent, during these times sugar bingers need to take extra precautions:

- ☆ Don't *make* candy, baked goods or sweets to give away as presents. Making sweet gifts is a guaranteed way to overeat. Instead, give non-food presents.

- ☆ When you're shopping, stay out of the candy aisles of the store so the sights and smells of the confections don't tempt you. If Halloween candy is a temptation to you, then give trick-or-treaters some non-food treats such as nickels (which cost less than most candy), or small, inexpensive plastic toys. Or pick a candy that you don't like and give that out.

- ☆ Similarly, if making an Easter basket for your children spells t-e-m-p-t-a-t-i-o-n or a chocolate binge, then make Easter sugar-free for the kids from now on. It's healthier all the way around to provide some non-food treats such as plastic eggs filled with money or toys. Or fill the baskets with healthful treats (provided they're not a binge food for you) such as nuts, raisins, trail mix or hard-boiled Easter eggs.

Birthdays are another difficult time for Yo-Yo Syndrome dieters because someone will invariably bake a cake. How do you turn down a slice of cake that someone has bought or made especially for you? There are several solutions:

- ☆ Let people know ahead of time that you choose not to eat any birthday cake. If you know they are going to buy or bake one for you, then politely tell them ahead of time, "Thank you but no thank you." I've found that this type of forewarning is appreciated, not resented. You could also suggest that the effort or money for the cake be used in other ways, such as for a light snack of fruit salad and frozen yogurt. You could even create a new birthday tradition—and reduce pressures to overeat—by offering to be the person who'll pick up the tab for a low-calorie birthday lunch.

  You could also (unless cake is your binge food), eat a few bites of the cake. After all, a few bites don't contain that many calories. Cake is only a problem if the sugar creates unsteady feelings in you, or if it is your binge food. After you take two or three bites, you could throw your crumpled napkin over the remaining cake to discourage yourself from eating any more.

  Or, you could do as one of my clients did and take the cake graciously. But then go into another room, with no one watching, and dispose of the cake slice (via garbage disposal or trash can). Then you can easily turn down a second slice.

Probably your best defence against automatic eating that's triggered when you go home for the holidays is to prepare for it. For example, recall how your eating behaviour changes when you go to your parents' (or other relatives') home. How can you plan to circumvent the pressure to eat there? If you're a Binge Eater, what steps can you take so that you won't eat your binge food while you're home?

- ☆ To avoid feeling like a little girl or boy (and thereby setting yourself up to overeat if you did so as a child), take some office or school work with you when you visit your parents. This "grown-up" material will provide a reminder of who you are as an adult; it will anchor you in the reality that you *are* an adult.

Emotion Eaters need to guard against stuffing feelings during the holidays and on birthdays. These emotionally volatile occasions, as mentioned before, are ripe for triggering overeating episodes. Feel yourself burning with anger at the way Uncle Ed talks to you? Upset because your sister's husband gave her diamonds for Christmas and you got a blender from your husband?

Worried because Dad's drinking too much brandy when his doctor told him to knock off the liquor? If you don't feel you can talk about it without causing a major family rift at a very inopportune time, then be sure to deal with your emotions in other ways. First, always admit your feelings to yourself instead of fighting or ignoring them. Second, go to a place where you can be alone (such as a bedroom, bathroom, the backyard or on a walk) or with a person who's non-judgmental and a good listener. Third, if you're alone, get your feelings out in the open by talking to your angels, God, Jesus, or whomever you feel spiritually attuned to. If you're with an empathetic listener, discuss your thoughts and feelings with this person (and say a prayer for spiritual support while you're at it, for good measure). Fourth, don't overeat because of your fattening feelings—it'll only make you feel worse!

If Christmas dinner means you'll be nibbling before and after the meal *plus* eating three servings of a huge turkey banquet, then consider the following:

☆ Why not eat at a restaurant next year? That way, you won't be "fat-igued" from cooking all day. In addition, there will be no temptation to nibble while cooking, and no leftovers to worry about.

☆ If you do eat Christmas dinner at home, be sure to chew sugarless gum while you're cooking. Sampling food and chewing gum are two activities, fortunately, that don't go together simultaneously. In addition, keep a glass of water or iced tea handy and drink it instead of picking at the turkey dressing or whatever else you're preparing.

☆ Plan ahead of time, as you normally do with all your meals, what you'll be eating for Christmas. Compose a personal menu that follows your Yo-Yo Diet Syndrome plan, and vow to stick to it no matter what. This plan reduces temptations to impulsively overeat.

Be sure to eat breakfast and lunch on Christmas Day. Starving before dinner serves no purpose other than to make you hungrier and more likely to overeat that night. If you're the host or hostess, serve yourself last during dinner, so that by the time you sit down to eat, others will have had time to make a substantial dent in their meals. That way, the smaller portions on your plate won't stand out as radically different from the amount of food others have.

If someone asks you why you're not returning for seconds, hold your stomach and dramatically say, "I'm absolutely stuffed! If I eat another bite, I'll explode!"

Remind yourself frequently that the true meaning of Christmas does not revolve around food. After dinner, send as many leftovers as you can home with guests to avoid overeating after dinner or the next day. If this isn't possible, then divide the leftovers into small portions and put them in the freezer immediately. You won't be as likely to overindulge if the food isn't readily accessible.

Many people postpone their diets during the holidays. This is especially true of the time period from the run-up to Christmas through to New Year, when people tend to let the eating floodgates loose. On New Year's Eve, they resolve to bring the overeating season to a halt. This is a practice that many seasonal Snowball Effect Eaters are particularly likely to engage in. If this habit seems familiar to you, remember that the Yo-Yo Diet Syndrome doesn't have a beginning or an ending. It is a way of life. Also keep in mind that your body doesn't take a holiday from converting fat and excess calories into body fat. It doesn't know whether today is your birthday or Christmas—it still gains or loses weight in the same way.

All in all, healing yourself from the Yo-Yo Diet Syndrome is an opportunity to shift your viewpoint of eating and food away from a belief that they constitute "entertainment", "recreation", "celebration", or "companionship". When food is no longer the focal point of holidays and birthdays, then human and spiritual interaction is the great centrepiece. Food often behaves as a wall that bars true intimacy with our family and our Higher Power. By removing that barrier, we may initially feel vulnerable, and fearful about getting close to others. However, that fear is soon replaced with love and true companionship.

Wedding Receptions

How many of you have gone to a wedding reception or a party and then spent the majority of the evening parked next to the snack table? I know I sure have.

In my therapy practice, I listened to more stories about overeating occurring at wedding receptions and parties than at any other place. And of these two, wedding receptions are definitely the number-one place where Yo-Yo Syndrome dieters overeat.

Many Yo-Yo Syndrome dieters run into fattening feelings at weddings. These may occur because you:

☆ feel left out, alone and awkward;

☆ worry that your weight will bar you from ever meeting Mr. or Ms. Right;

☆ wish that you had a romantic life like the bride and groom;

☆ believe that no one's paying attention to you;

☆ are jealous that the bride is getting all the attention and gifts;

☆ become aware of the contrast between your marriage and that of the bride-to-be's; and

☆ feel uncomfortable about being around inebriated people and in close proximity to acquaintances or relatives whom you may not care for.

> Sally, for example, had been healing herself from the Yo-Yo Diet Syndrome for four months when she was invited to her cousin's wedding. The wedding was at a huge resort, and the bride's parents spent a fortune on catering, flowers and the wedding dress. Sally was envious of the money and attention her cousin, the bride, was getting. But at the same time, Sally felt guilt for being "petty". Sally also didn't know quite how to act

> at so regal an affair and felt very uncomfortable and self-conscious. She didn't know whether to fold her arms or keep her hands in her pockets as she stood at the wedding reception.
>
> "Everyone else seems so sure of themselves," Sally said to herself. "They all fit in here, but I don't!" Feeling left out and despondent, Sally headed toward the buffet table even though she knew the food would tempt her. She looked at the chocolate torte with the delicate roses frosted on each slice and thought, "One of those would make me feel better. I've lost 15 pounds for this wedding and no one even noticed it. Just one piece of cake won't hurt me. No one will know...no one will even care!"
>
> Before she could talk herself out of it, Sally had the torte in her mouth and was lovingly, almost sensuously, appreciating its creaminess. Too quickly, it was gone, and Sally unhappily grabbed another slice. Sally felt nauseated with sugar and chocolate by the time she pulled herself away from the remaining slices of cake. Counting what was left—had she really eaten that many?—Sally felt disgusted with herself.

A wedding is an emotionally charged situation. It's very draining, whether you're in the audience or in the wedding party. So the abundance of food often spells trouble for the Yo-Yo Syndrome dieter who's in an emotional upheaval about the whole event. What can Yo-Yo Syndrome dieters do to avoid overeating at weddings?

First, stay as far away from snack and buffet tables as you can. It's just too tempting to endlessly snack as a way of handling your fattening feelings. Instead, keep your hands full by holding a glass of sparkling water or by offering to help the bride's parents with any last-minute details such as arranging the wedding gifts or table centrepieces.

If you're holding the wedding at your own house, you'll need to be particularly alert to avoid overeating in response to anxiety and pressures. My client Jo, for instance, overate when she held a wedding reception at her house because she was so worried that the guests wouldn't approve of the job she had done in decorating and catering. It's also nerve-wracking to go to a wedding where you don't know any of the other guests. Jeannie, another client of mine, accompanied her new boyfriend to a wedding where she didn't know anyone. Because she felt so self-conscious and awkward ("I didn't feel like I dressed right for the occasion, and it was like I was all thumbs the entire day—meanwhile, my boyfriend was having a great time with all his old friends"), Jeannie stood by the snack table all evening to appear busy. She ended up going on an all-out eating binge.

A second way to avoid overeating at weddings is to go out of your way to mingle with other guests. If you're uncomfortable because, like Jeannie, you don't know anyone at the affair, look for someone else who seems lonely and start a conversation by asking an open-ended question (one that can't be answered with a mere yes or no) such as, "How long have you known Tom and Mary?" "Where do you live?" or "What time is the band supposed to start playing?"

Third, if you have some fattening feelings before, during or after the wedding, remember that you can choose not to attend the wedding reception. Or you can decide only to make a very brief appearance.

Parties and Get-Togethers

Parties, although meant to be fun occasions, can at times be extremely stressful, particularly if you're feeling fat and uncomfortable about the way you look, feeling awkward with the people around you, feeling invisible—as if you don't matter to anyone— or the opposite, feeling as if everyone's staring at you and judging you. All these feelings can send you to the chip-and-dip bowl, where you're apt to munch away your anguish instead of dealing with it.

There can also be pressure to eat at parties. A friend of mine, for instance, throws the most elaborate affairs. The trouble is, they all revolve around food and eating. As you walk into his house, the first sight you see is a giant oak table in an elevated dining room. The table is practically buckling under the weight of dozens of sterling-silver platters, bowls and pitchers—all containing the most aesthetically appealing food you've ever seen. Guests spend most of the evening wandering around the table looking at the food, eating the food, and talking about the food. At parties such as this, it's difficult to *not overeat* and remain inconspicuous.

However, instead of avoiding the company of my friend and the other guests, I've learned to follow these guidelines so I can have a good time and also eat light:

☆ The first and most important rule for eating light at non-dinner parties is to eat your meal before going to the party. Make it a leisurely meal, complete with plenty of liquids to fill you up. Decide beforehand that you won't be eating anything at the party.

☆ Arrive fashionably late. In this way, the others will have already eaten so you won't feel any pressure to join in.

☆ Carry a glass of sparkling water, complete with a wedge of lemon or lime, in your hand. This will reduce the risk of feeling awkwardly empty-handed, as well as prevent others from pushing plates of food into your hands.

- ☆ If the party is a potluck, picnic or barbecue, bring a low-calorie and healthful dish such as a colourful vegetable tray or fresh-fruit salad. That way, if you become extra-hungry, you'll have something to munch on that won't sabotage your weight-loss efforts.

- ☆ If you feel the urge to eat, quickly offer to help the host or hostess with party details. Pour drinks for other guests, fold napkins, take arriving guests' coats or drive to the convenience store for some forgotten party necessity. Just do something other than eat!

- ☆ If you have any fattening feelings such as anger, embarrassment or jealousy, go into the nearest rest room or go outside alone. Close your eyes for a few moments, and take three deep breaths. Tell yourself something comforting such as: "I'm a good person" or "I like myself." Pray for spiritual support and guidance. Give yourself a mental hug, and when you feel composed, return to the party.

- ☆ If you're not having a good time, or if you feel out of control with your appetite, then excuse yourself and leave the party. People leave parties early all the time; give yourself permission to do so if you need to.

Keeping Up the Diet at Work

Whether it's a cafeteria, the pastry cart, the co-worker's candy dish or the vending machine down the hall, temptations to overeat abound at the workplace. What's a Yo-Yo Syndrome dieter, bent on avoiding overeating, supposed to do? Let me tell you about some of the ingenious solutions my working clients have come up with over the years:

Katherine keeps a pretty bowl of naturally sweetened and flavoured sugar-free hard candies and gum on her desk. She says that by keeping her mouth busy with sugarless treats, she keeps her mind off the fattening foods her co-workers indulge in.

Patty was upset because there was always an open box of doughnuts in the office lounge. Every time she'd take a break, the doughnuts would be right there staring her in the face. Now she throws a big towel over the box when she's on break— kind of an "out-of-sight, out-of-mind" solution.

Sonya, who was faced with the same dilemma, solved it by talking with her co-workers and requesting that they keep the doughnut box up on a shelf where it was still accessible to others but out of Sonya's immediate sight.

Similarly, Hope worked in the back office of a store and had a desk that faced a giant display of cookies. Every day, Hope stared at the cookies and sometimes did more than stare—she ate them! To conquer this problem, Hope finally had to change to a desk across the room.

Bridget's dilemma was that every time she'd get frustrated at work, she'd stomp away from her desk and head for the candy-vending machine.

Now that she's been healing herself from the Yo-Yo Diet Syndrome for three months, Bridget stomps off to the juice machine and buys a bottle of apple juice.

Margie, another client who was hooked on vending-machine candy and chips, found that there was only one way to keep herself away from this junk food: she stopped bringing any money to work.

Dianna solved the same problem in a different way. She explained to her close friends at work that she was trying to lose weight, and asked if they would please help her when she was about to break her diet. Luckily, Dianna's co-workers are good friends (you wouldn't want to make such a request to just anybody!), because they've given her support at times when she was just about to overeat. "Twice I've been walking down the hall toward the vending machines," Dianna told me, "and my friends have run up to me and said, 'Oh, no, you don't, Dianna! You're not going to break your diet now, not after you've lost this much weight!'" While we all have to take responsibility for our own eating, having support from others at work is definitely helpful.

Another client, Leigh, convinced her employer to start an exercise programme for employees. The employer got Leigh and her co-workers a special group rate at a local gym, and this spurred many people in the company to become weight- and health-conscious. Now, instead of sitting around eating pastries all day, the co-workers exchange diet tips and go to the gym together after work.

Mary has learned to schedule her work day so that she's busy when her co-workers are snacking. While she still eats lunch with others, Mary plans her breaks so that the mobile-snack coach is not around when she leaves her desk.

Sarah has found that she eats less and feels more satisfied if, after eating her lunch, she takes a brisk walk around the high school where she teaches. Lately, she's been walking with another health-conscious teacher, and it appears that Sarah has found herself a new friend in the process.

Tiffany was so fed up with having desserts pushed at her and left on her desk by co-workers that she decided to bring in a pepper shaker and keep it in her desk. Now, whenever a co-worker won't take no for an answer and insists on giving Tiffany some food, she pours pepper on it. This renders it inedible and removes the temptation for her to overeat her binge food.

Another client, Angela, had to admit to herself that she was encouraging her co-workers to push fattening goodies on her. Angela was unwittingly giving her co-workers a lot of attention every time she'd protest at their offers of candy or cookies.

Elaine always seemed to be in a quandary on her lunch hour—would it better for her to eat lunch or run errands? There never seemed to be enough time to do both, and that meant that Elaine would often skip lunch and overeat at dinnertime. Finally, Elaine had to examine her priorities. She clearly saw that skipping lunch was not a viable option for her if she wanted to maintain her weight loss. So Elaine has learned to run errands after work and on weekends.

Tom found that he'd unintentionally overeat when he worked through his lunch hour. To halt this tendency, Tom made a strict pact with himself to not eat at his desk.

Ruth, a Stress Eater, would overeat when she'd take potential clients out to lunch. Finally, she had to figure out a way to curtail this tendency without hurting her business. She's found that using meditation techniques before a business lunch calms her nerves. She also limits her business lunches to one particular restaurant near her office where light yet great-tasting food is served.

The cafeteria at the hospital where Jan works rarely serves food that fits into her diet plan. Although it seems surprising that a medical institution would serve unhealthy food, most of the food at the employee cafeteria consists of fatty meats covered with buttery sauces. To stay on her eating plan, Jan had to bring her own lunches to work—something that requires extra planning, but was worthwhile in terms of Jan's success with her weight and eating. Now, she sometimes brings a light frozen meal to work and microwaves it. Other times, she'll prepare a healthful chef's salad and keep it in the hospital kitchen's cafeteria until lunchtime.

Lisa couldn't stomach eating breakfast before going to work (she leaves home at 6:00 a.m.). She used to skip breakfast, but ever since she's begun her new diet plan, she has been making both her breakfast and lunch at night and bringing them to work with her the next day.

Audrey worked the 11:00 p.m. to 7:00 a.m. shift at a factory, and she found that the graveyard shift was not at all helpful in breaking out of her Yo-Yo Diet Syndrome. It seemed that Audrey was always confused about what time of day it was, and she never knew whether it was time for breakfast, lunch or dinner (kind of like me when I travel to different time zones on an airplane). "I wake up at 9:00 p.m. to get ready for work and eat my first meal of the day," Audrey explained. "Now, is that my breakfast because it's my first meal, or is it my dinner because I'm eating at 9:00 at night?" Unfortunately, this confusion often meant that Audrey ate too much food, too many times a day. She'd also go right to sleep after eating in the late morning hours. Finally, Audrey had to admit that her graveyard shift was spelling the death of her dieting efforts. Her solution was to get transferred to the first shift (7:00 a.m. to 3:00 p.m.), and in this way, she was able to stick to her diet plan and have three meals a day.

Carol learned not to tell her co-workers that she was watching her weight. "When I'd say I was eating lighter, it was like I was a Buckingham Palace guard—the way they spent all their time taunting me and trying to tempt me with food so I'd overeat!" Once she kept this news to herself, her co-workers left her alone.

On Spouses, Lovers, Relatives and Friends

Carol's situation at work with taunting, teasing, and tempting co-workers is probably similar to reactions you may have received while watching your weight. What do you do when you're trying to lose weight and one of the following happens to you?

- ☆ Your spouse begins to bring home boxes of your favourite desserts.
- ☆ Your mother insists that you try the cake she baked just for you.
- ☆ Your best friend says you look gaunt and "way too thin" (even though you know your weight is still too heavy for your height and build).

☆ Your sister asks for details about your diet plan, then proceeds to list reason after reason why "it'll never work for you".

☆ Your boyfriend tells you he likes the way you look now and insists he doesn't find trim women attractive.

Quite likely, you've met with these and similar situations that have either triggered discomfort or proven to be a catalyst for overeating. It's also probable that you'll have encounters like these in the future, so it's best to prepare for them in advance. This doesn't mean being defensive or carrying a chip on your shoulder— just having a few tools ready in case you need them.

As I mentioned in Chapter Six (on Self-Esteem Eaters), it's important for you to understand exactly why you want to lose weight. If you're trying to slim down to elicit compliments from your spouse or lover, then you've given him or her too much power over your weight. You'll become discouraged when he or she doesn't notice the ten pounds you lost, and you'll feel you've been given "permission" to overeat if your lover gives you chocolate candies or some other gift of food.

To maintain a healthy figure, the only motivating force that works is *losing weight to please yourself.* Unless you have the distorted mental body image that accompanies the eating disorder anorexia nervosa, you must adhere to your own standards of what weight feels best on you. If someone says you look like a skeleton and you are still above what the standard weight charts recommend for your height and build, then disregard the comment. Phrases such as, "If you lose any more weight, you'll blow away" are meant to be flattering compliments, not a standard to determine whether to overeat or not.

If people are pushy in their "you're too thin" admonishments, you can handle the situation in one of several ways. You can pretend you didn't hear them and change the subject, or remain silent. You can thank them for the compliment and then change the subject. You can say, "Thanks for your concern, but I know what weight I feel healthiest with. If I need some feedback in the future, I'll be sure to ask you for it." Or you can use a stronger phrase (after repeated attempts to get the person to knock it off) such as, "I feel distressed that you don't seem to hear me when I ask you to back off about my weight. I'm really starting to resent the intrusions, and I'm afraid if you don't stop, it will hurt our relationship."

But what about people who push food under your nose, sending delicate aromas directly into your brain's appetite centre? What about the man who teased you three months ago about the size of your behind, but who is now offering you bites of his candy bar? And how about your poor mother, who seemingly slaved to create the fattening dessert she's now tempting you with? Could you ever live with yourself again if you turned her down? What if something happened to her tomorrow and you hadn't honoured her last request to you?

What do you do in these admittedly slippery and emotionally fraught situations? If you know you're likely to encounter a "diet saboteur", then your best bet is to psych yourself up the same way you would for any challenging situation, such as asking your boss for a raise.

As you're getting dressed to go to Mum's for dinner, mentally rehearse how you will keep your eating in check for the evening. Remember, you are an adult and how you eat is your business and nobody else's! When you say no to someone's offering, you are not rejecting that person (which is the thought that triggers the fattening feeling of guilt); you are merely rejecting the food in his or her hands.

Try to put yourself in the other person's shoes to understand what is motivating him or her to push food on you. Everyone's not out to get you, even though it can feel that way at times. For example, one client complained that her husband brought home her favourite doughnuts every night. At first, she was furious that he could be so insensitive, but upon looking more closely at her situation, we found that she was actually *rewarding* her husband for bringing home treats. She'd act very happy, agreeable and loving the whole time she was eating the doughnuts. This attitude encouraged her husband to bring home the pastries each evening.

So, be assertive and spell out exactly how you feel about someone's food-pushing. Assertiveness, unlike aggressiveness, means that you have regard for the other person's emotions while you talk about your *own* feelings. For instance, an aggressive person would say, "I'm so angry at you for bringing home those damn cookies when I've asked you not to! How could you be so inconsiderate?" An assertive person, in contrast, would phrase the same feelings in a way that would permit communication, because defensiveness would be kept to a minimum. A better way of expressing anger might sound something like this: "I need to tell you that I feel exasperated right now. I am trying really hard to lose weight, and it's a very difficult thing to do. What I need right now more than anything is your support, and that means not bringing tubs of ice cream home with you at night. I really mean this—it's important to me that you stop."

When Others Act Jealous

> Roberta came into my office and started crying. "I feel so guilty!" she sobbed. "My husband is sure that I'm going to have an affair now that I've lost the weight, and I hate to see him so upset and worried." Roberta had no intention of cheating on her husband, but she also didn't want his jealousy to disrupt their relationship. She was even considering putting her weight back on just to regain peace in her house. Fortunately, she realized that she'd be miserable if she were overweight

> again, and that her husband's distrust reflected his own poor self-image, and not her own.

Roberta's spouse, like many husbands, did initially feel threatened when his wife transformed into a svelte beauty. He felt insecure, as if he were unworthy of being married to such an attractive woman. Surely, he thought, she would now leave him for a man befitting her.

Often, time heals a spouse's insecurities. When your husband, boyfriend, wife or girlfriend sees that you are not going to leave, he or she will relax. If not, you will have to look at your own behaviour next to be certain you are not provoking the jealousy (by openly flirting in front of him or her, or by dressing very provocatively). If you aren't engaged in potentially threatening behaviour, then you'll need to conclude that your lover has personal insecurity. You may not be able to change him or her into a secure person. Deep insecurity—the kind that doesn't respond to reassurances from others—often has its roots in earlier experiences with rejection (from parents or a first love, for example) and has little to do with you.

Since healing the Yo-Yo Diet Syndrome involves much more than merely cutting down on fats and calories, your change in lifestyle could have temporarily upset the balance in your relationship. Many of my clients who, as part of their healing process, went back to school or changed careers, found that their spouses and families sometimes showed concern. Changes of any kind, even positive ones, may require an adjustment period for your loved ones to get used to your new lifestyle. This is especially the case when you've made radical and sudden modifications in your behaviour and schedule.

Your best bet in dealing with a spouse or lover who displays jealousy is an honest exchange of feelings about one another. You can begin such a talk by sharing your own deep feelings. Choose a quiet moment when you're alone together and won't be interrupted for a while, and begin with something such as: "I feel that there have been some changes in the way we relate to one another lately. It all seems to have happened since I lost weight. It really upsets me, too, and I wonder if we could discuss it." Avoid hurling accusations or saying something like, "You seem so jealous lately," as this is apt to be met with defensiveness and denial.

The response to your opening statement will likely sound something like, "Yeah, I know there have been some changes. *You* sure have changed since you lost the weight!"

Even though your jaw may drop at this moment, resist the impulse to defensively say, "Me? You think *I'm* the one who's changed?!" Instead, ask your lover for more information to get to the heart of his or her jealousy: "In what ways do you believe that I've changed?" You may be surprised by the answer, but you'll probably also hear some truths.

At this point, lovingly share all of your feelings. Tell your partner what being fit and changing your life means to you. Talk about how exciting your life is now, and how you'd like to see your lover work on some life-enriching goals, too. And most of all, reassure your lover that all of these changes do not spell rejection. You are not leaving him or her—you're just shedding your fattening and unhealthy lifestyle.

Again, it may take time for your partner to adjust to the new you. Stick with your new diet plan, though, and don't go back to your old eating and lifestyle habits no matter how jealous the other person becomes. No one is worth your being unfit again. Not only lovers act jealous, though. Your platonic friends may become envious when your body starts to slim down. As a result, you may experience fears of rejection, abandonment, anger at their conditional love, and hurt at being excluded.

> At first Charlotte thought she was imagining being excluded from the get-togethers that her small circle of friends customarily engaged in.

"For years, Harry and I would meet with three other couples for drinks, dinner or card games," Charlotte told me. "We were all really close and enjoyed each other's company tremendously!" That is, until Charlotte lost 30 pounds.

"I had always been struggling with my weight," she explained, "but I'd been heavy since these people had known me. When I decided to eat lighter, they were all so supportive! They complimented me on the way I looked each time they saw me, and after I got the whole 30 pounds off, they made me feel like a princess. I mean, a couple of the husbands in the group kept staring at me all evening." Charlotte's eyes turned downward. "It's painful to think about—and I think it really sounds vain of me—but I'm sure that two of the gals in our group are threatened by my new figure, and that's why they haven't invited Harry and me to the get-togethers for the past month."

Another client, Sandra, was also stinging from the rejection connected to her weight loss. Her circle of friends had consisted of five other women she'd known from church, who went out to lunch twice a week together. They'd eat enormous meals, complete with dessert, and spend hours talking about their kids, their husbands and life in general.

When Sandra first began to lose weight, the others teased her with, "Aw, you'll never do it!" gibes. Then, as Sandra continued to eat small lunches and pass up dessert, the comments turned into cold shoulders. "I could feel that they were sore at me," Sandra remembered. "It was like I

> was violating some code of ethics by not overeating with them." The group's attitude became so uncomfortable for Sandra that she began missing the lunch dates and avoiding the group members at church. The ensuing feelings of loneliness and betrayal almost sent Sandra back to overeating more than a few times.

When a friend signals jealousy over your weight loss, it's important to remember a few things. First, the bad feelings your friend is experiencing aren't coming from you—they're coming from that person's ego. I remember one summer when I was carrying 35 extra pounds on my body. It was a hot summer, and I spent a lot of time at my sister-in-law's swimming pool, where we had a great time splashing about (she and I were both overweight). Some days, though, her cousin—a tall, thin clothes horse—would join us at the pool. Between her body and her wardrobe, I remember feeling as if I despised that woman. She was a very nice person and never did one mean thing to me, but when I saw her I felt bad about myself. And instead of acknowledging those feelings, I transferred them onto her.

In spiritual truth, our higher self—as well as a friend's—is incapable of feeling or expressing jealousy, since this emotion is based in a belief in lack and the thought, "If one person wins, the other person loses." Our higher selves know no such thing as loss or competition, so focus on the truth of your friend and the situation, and release any guilt your ego may try to foist upon you.

If your "jealous" friends have always been close to you, then have a heart-to-heart talk with them just as you would with a spouse or lover, as described earlier. And remember, a real friend will love you whether you're fat or fit. If someone rejects you because of what you look like, he or she wasn't that close of a friend to begin with.

Finally, if the jealous friend was an acquaintance, then maybe it's time to let go of the relationship. You don't need to waste precious moments of your life trying to please someone who doesn't have your best interests at heart. And if this person triggers fattening feelings in you, you especially need to avoid him or her.

Aesop first said it, and it's now a cliché, but it's so true and especially appropriate in this discussion on dealing with others: *Please all, and you will please no one.* Losing weight and getting fit are not a thoughtless act that can hurt someone you care about. It's not selfish in the usual sense of the word. Therefore, it's illogical for others to treat you poorly just because you've lost weight. While it's wise to understand their point of view, don't let anyone step on you either. Take good care of yourself through your new diet plan, and be your own best friend.

Ending on a Friendly Note

Not everyone will have ulterior motives or be jealous as you lose weight. Some social obstacles are created by practical sources. Think for a moment about when and where you normally see your friends. Chances are you'll answer, "When we eat dinner together." Many people who diet give up these social gatherings and, along with them, the chance to be with their friends.

However, there are lots of ways to maintain your social network and not invite temptation to overeat. Among them:

- ☆ Have a light party! Why not throw a party for you and your friends and serve healthful foods and beverages? Even your friends who aren't health-conscious will appreciate the opportunity to get together and will enjoy your lighter fare.

  Parties can also revolve around some activity other than eating. How about a horseshoe throw or a swimming party? Why not organize a painting party, where everyone comes dressed in their grubbies and pitches in to get a whole house painted in an afternoon? Offer organized games such as charades for your guests, or hire a band and clear the floor for some calorie-burning dancing. How about a sing-along around the piano? (Sounds corny, I know, but it is really enjoyable!) At a party with a non-food theme, you and your guests will have fun and welcome the change from stuffy sit-down dinner parties.

☆ Exercise with your friends. Don't see much of your friends now that you don't go out to lunch with them any more? Why not invite one or two of them to go the gym or yoga class with you? Or, for her birthday, buy your best friend a one-month, half-year or full-year membership at the gym you attend.

☆ Another great idea is to form a walking group. Decide on a time and meeting place, and then go for long walks with your friends. This will give you lots of time to catch up on the latest news, expose you to fresh air and pretty scenery, and help burn those calories.

☆ Go clothes shopping with your friends. Whether you buy, window-shop or just try on different styles, clothes shopping is a good way to stay inspired to attain or maintain a fit body. Shopping with friends can also turn an average shopping day into a fun adventure.

☆ Sign up for a class with a friend. Have you ever had a secret yearning to learn how to make stained glass, go windsurfing, learn psychic development or improve your photography skills? Chances are that one or two of your

> friends have, too. Why not check the schedule of the local adult school, the parks and recreation department, the bookstore or the community college nearest you? After gathering the necessary information, urge your interested friends to enrol with you. Not only will you get to spend time together in an activity that doesn't involve food, but you'll also have fun and learn new skills.

Losing weight doesn't have to mean isolating yourself from people whose company you enjoy. You still can eat lunch or dinner together, after all, as long as you stick with your eating plan. I think you'll find that the longer you stay on your new diet plan, the more you'll want to spend your free time playing, learning and generally being active. You won't want to spend all your time eating any more!

CHAPTER TWELVE

WEIGHT MAINTENANCE AND THE LAST FEW POUNDS

"Set your mind on things above, not on things on the earth."

—Apostle Paul, Col. 3:2

There's no better time than now to have a fit, healthful body. After all, how many more summers do you want to slip by before you get into shape? At how many more holiday parties do you want to feel uncomfortably overweight? How about high-school reunions? Wouldn't you love to feel toned and trim at your next one?

And even more important, wouldn't you like to feel great about your life? Wouldn't you like to wake up in the morning and feel excited as you look forward to the day's events? There's no better time to begin healing your entire life than today. Face it, tomorrow will be pretty much like today. There's no reason *not* to start taking steps toward transforming your life and your body—NOW!

If, during the days that follow, you do happen to slip up and overeat, please don't give up on yourself. Please don't kick yourself or say, "I'm a failure." Such negative talk only leads into the downward emotional spirals that keep you overeating. My mother, who is a recovering Yo-Yo Syndrome dieter, always points out a great way of demonstrating this:

Let's say you're driving from your house to the airport. You accidentally get off at the wrong exit. At that point, you don't just keep driving down the wrong road, do you? No! As soon as you realize the error that you've made, you simply get right back on the road until you find the correct exit ramp.

Well, that's exactly how it is with the Yo-Yo Diet Syndrome, too. If, for any reason, you find yourself overeating, follow the suggestions below to immediately get yourself back on the road toward your destination. Don't keep driving on the wrong road of an eating binge.

☆ Know that all guilt feelings connected to overeating stem from your ego. Your guilt is not a sign that you are bad or weak-willed in any way. Rather, it's a sign that your ego knows that your higher self is taking over. When that happens, your ego fights for its very life in any way possible. Your ego will orchestrate fattening feelings designed to trigger an overeating episode and, having done so, will then proceed to viciously berate you for overeating. Combat this cycle by refusing to listen to your ego at all. Instead, ask for spiritual support that will remind you of the beautiful, strong and capable being who you are in truth.

☆ Call a supportive friend. Talk with this person about your eating, and ask for emotional support as you get back on track.

☆ Go to an Overeaters Anonymous meeting. While you're there, it's very important that you talk to the group about your slip-up even though it may feel frightening, humiliating or humbling. After you talk about it, you'll receive lots of understanding and healthy, appropriate support from group members. This will renew your commitment and belief in yourself.

- ☆ Reread this book for additional reinforcement and support.
- ☆ Destroy any binge foods you have in your home, office, purse or car. Don't wait to "give them away to a neighbour" or offer some other excuse—get rid of them now!

Although I don't wish a slip-up on anybody, I do want to acknowledge that sometimes it is the best thing that can happen to someone. Let me explain. I was seeing a new client, Brian, because his mother Debra had done well on her recovery from the Yo-Yo Diet Syndrome, and she knew that her son needed this particular brand of help as well.

> Brian, a 22-year-old college student, came to therapy reluctantly. He knew he wanted help with his excess weight, but he wasn't sure how a psychotherapist was going to be able to help him. Still, he kept reminding himself how much weight his mother had lost on my programme. As I explained the concept of binge foods to Brian, he immediately told me that he knew his were salty junk foods. When I told him then about abstinence as one way of preventing eating binges, I could see that Brian didn't quite buy my theory. He agreed to try it anyway, and for the next month he stayed away from salty junk foods completely. He even lost 11 pounds in the process.
>
> Then Brian had to go out of state for one of his college courses. While he was away from all the reminders of his Yo-Yo Diet Syndrome, he ate his binge food, starting with one bag of potato crisps. This sent Brian into a full-blown eating binge that lasted until he returned home two months later and made an appointment with me.

> When I saw Brian, I knew that he was now convinced he was a Binge Eater. He had experienced firsthand an eating binge triggered by one bite of his binge food, and since he had gained knowledge and insight about his Yo-Yo Diet Syndrome, he knew exactly what he had to do. Because of his slip, Brian had completely accepted that he needed to abstain from his binge food forever—a day at a time.

And that's why slips can sometimes be beneficial. Before his slip, Brian was staying away from salty junk food purely to please me and his mother. Following his eating binge, however, Brian's motivation became completely internal—he was abstaining because he was absolutely sure there was no such thing as just one bite. This internal motivation makes all the difference when recovering from the Yo-Yo Diet Syndrome.

Those Last Few Pounds

Most of us know the struggle of losing those final five to ten pounds before reaching a comfortable weight and fitness level. Up until that point, your weight may have come off with relative ease; now you come to a grinding halt as you get closer and closer to your final destination. At this point, you may become frustrated and overwhelmed. Some people even decide to stay at the weight they've landed at, making that their goal weight. And that's certainly okay as long as you're happy at the weight and body-fat percentage you've reached. If you're satisfied with the weight your body naturally veers toward, then that's what counts.

If, however, you really do want to shave off those extra few pounds or fat percentage points, then here are some tips that can help push you over the plateau edge to your goal:

☆ Intensify your exercise programme. If you're now exercising four days a week, you may need to work out five days for a while to get those last stubborn pounds off. If you're in the beginner's step-aerobics class, you may need to move to the intermediate level. If you're walking half a mile a day, try one mile of faster walking for a while.

☆ Keep your focus on today, and stay positively motivated. Don't look at your weight loss negatively ("Oh, my gosh, I've only lost ten pounds since I started this diet. I've got over ten more pounds to lose. I'll never get there!") because you'll end up discouraged and overwhelmed. Instead, focus on one pound at a time. Take a "can do" approach ("Great! I've lost two pounds since Wednesday. Now I'll focus on losing two more pounds. My energy is high, my muscles feel toned, and I feel terrific!"), and you'll find that your motivation stays high, and your progress and weight loss will be satisfying.

☆ Remember to visualize yourself at your goal fitness level so that your behaviour matches your self-image. If you see yourself as unfit, you will eat and exercise as an unfit person. If you see yourself as fit, you will naturally eat lighter and at a slower pace. You will put your heart into your workout programme. And, as Ralph Waldo Emerson so wisely put it, "We are what we think about all day long."

☆ Increase your water intake. Barring health restrictions (such as some cardiovascular or kidney disorders, which your doctor should advise you about), you can never drink too much water! Water also has an amazing way of getting people off weight plateaus. If you're drinking one half gallon a day now, then try drinking one gallon instead, and see if that doesn't "tip the scales" for you.

The side benefits of a clearer complexion and decreased appetite also make drinking plenty of water a good idea.

- ☆ Cut out red meats entirely until you reach your goal weight. I've had clients whose weight wouldn't budge until they took this step and eliminated beef and pork from their diets. If you are at a plateau, maybe this would be a good idea for you, too.

- ☆ Some Yo-Yo Syndrome dieters may need to cut out snack eating, especially late in the evening. Many clients get great results from eating their dinners earlier in the evening, so they have time to digest before bedtime.

- ☆ Refuse to give up! No matter how frustrating a fitness plateau is, don't let it get the best of you. Besides, it would be illogical to gain all the weight back and lose your muscle tone just because you're momentarily frustrated. If you follow the steps involved in healing yourself from the Yo-Yo Diet Syndrome, the weight and fat will come off. You may be accustomed to fad diets that rapidly took the pounds off, so it's important to remember that this programme is different, in that weight loss will be a bit slower. "Quickie" diets just don't result in permanent weight loss or established changes in eating behaviour in the way that balanced, realistic and more moderate modifications do.

Maintaining Your Fitness

You've done it! You've reached your goal fitness level and you look and feel fantastic. Even though you've probably been fit like this before, this time you're going to *stay* fit. I remember the last time I lost all my excess weight. I was happy, of course, but I also expected to start putting all the weight back on again. I was so accustomed to gaining weight immediately after losing it that it actually felt odd to keep the weight off. Just as your equilibrium makes you feel as though you're still swaying in the waves after stepping off a rocking boat onto firm ground, I felt a strong momentum to keep going with my past pattern of gaining and losing, losing and gaining. But I was also determined to try to keep it off this time. I say "try" because, since I'd never experienced long-term weight maintenance, I wasn't exactly sure I was capable of it. My only hope, I knew, was to keep taking my diet one day at a time. And I used many of the tips that are outlined in this book. Believe me, I needed all the help I could get.

Since everyone is so different, only you will know how much food you can eat and how much exercise to do and still successfully maintain or improve your present fitness level. The key elements to consider in deciding what fitness level is right for you can come from asking yourself:

Do I feel that I have enough energy throughout the day? Do I wake up feeling refreshed? Do I feel alert throughout the day? Am I able to concentrate on important tasks? Does it seem that I have approximately the same amount (or more) of vim and vigour as other people? Do my moods stay fairly stable? Do I rarely or never feel light-headed or dizzy? Do I rarely or never suffer from exercise-related injuries? Do my friends and family rarely or never complain that I'm not eating enough? Do my friends or family rarely or never complain that I exercise too much?

If you answered no to two or more of these questions, something is wrong, and your diet and exercise programme may be the culprit.

The point of recovering from the Yo-Yo Diet Syndrome is to enable you to attain and maintain a fitness level that promotes good mental, physical and spiritual health. However, if you overdo it and eat too little, eat non-nutritious meals, exercise too vigorously or don't drink enough water, then your energy level, concentration and moods will suffer.

There is no good reason to slash your food intake or to overdo your workout programme. There is no "thinness competition" that you must win, and very few potential romantic partners will be attracted to a person who is gaunt, surly and spaced-out. Your fitness goal isn't about what size jeans you can wear but, more important, how much energy and excitement you have in your life. You want to be able to focus and concentrate, so you'll naturally choose healthful foods that are both light and nutritious. Since you want to be even-tempered, you'll eat three healthful meals a day. You want to feel great when you wake up in the morning, so you'll be sure to only put positive foods into your mouth, and positive thoughts into your mind.

If You Gain Weight...

It's almost impossible to stay at exactly the same weight without some minor fluctuations, usually brought on by fluid retention (especially during menstrual cycles). This is the same as when you drive your car down a perfectly straight road—you tend to move the steering wheel ever so slightly.

Therefore, please don't berate yourself for normal weight swings. Such negative self-talk can undo all the improvements you've worked so hard to make. What you want to avoid—at all costs—are the sharp veers that would send you off the road and into a ditch. Memorize this, please: *No More Yo-Yoing*. Hang up a sign if you like, with a picture of a yo-yo in a red circle with a big red NO slash across it.

However, since yo-yoing is a lifestyle habit, it is possible that you may unwittingly allow your weight to creep up. If that happens, it's important to first uncover the source of the regained weight by asking yourself the following questions about common causes of weight gain:

☆ "Did I gain weight after recently eating at a restaurant?" If so, then you probably had too big a meal or food that was high in sodium (such as MSG used at Asian restaurants or salted chips at Mexican restaurants). Plan to avoid that restaurant, eat a much smaller meal there the next time, or ask that the food be prepared without salt or MSG.

☆ "Did I gain the weight from making my portions too big?" Some people who are wary of the "one serving only" guideline in this book pile two helpings onto their plate and call it "one serving". Please be honest with yourself when you are eating, and watch the portion size on your plate.

☆ "Did I gain weight from eating foods high in fat, calories, and/or sodium?" Perhaps you're using whole milk instead of skim or low-fat, or are eating marbled red meats, fried meats or fish, or cheese and cream-based sauces. If so, a few healthful adjustments to your menu can undo your weight gain.

☆ "Did I gain weight from not exercising enough?" If you've let your fitness programme slip, you'll be burning calories at a slower rate, probably retaining water, and possibly overeating due to fatigue from a sedentary lifestyle. Recommit yourself to physical fitness, and you'll kick-start your overall wellness.

☆ "Did I gain the weight from skipping meals?" If you skip meals, your body won't burn calories as efficiently, and you're likely to overeat at the following meal. If you're doing "creative dieting", it will be helpful to reread Chapter Nine.

☆ "Did I gain the weight from eating my binge food?" Binge Eaters who eat their binge food will find that their appetite for all foods increases. For this very important reason, consider abstaining from your binge food.

☆ "Did I gain the weight after eating large snacks?" Are your after-dinner snacks an endless feast of finger foods? If so, then you may be someone who cannot snack. Some people are just unable to stop eating after they have a snack. These folks need to have their snacks immediately after lunch and dinner, then brush their teeth and stick to non-calorific fluids (such as sparkling water or herbal tea) until it's time for their next meal.

☆ "Did I gain the weight from retaining water?" If you're not drinking eight glasses of water a day, chances are that your weight gain stems from fluid retention. This is especially true if you're eating foods high in sodium or are drinking more than two diet colas a day. It's important to keep your water intake high in order to flush out excess salt and water.

You Can Do It!

No matter what you've been told in the past, no matter what negative beliefs you've held about yourself, you really *can* have a fit body. It doesn't matter how old you are, how much money you do or don't have, how many years you went to school, what your love life is or has been like, how many children you've had, or anything else—you can get fit now and stay fit for good!

Keep in mind that every time you pick up your fork or spoon, you are engaged in the process of making a choice. You are choosing, at that moment, your fitness level. If you overeat or indulge in fattening foods, your body's weight will be heavier. If you eat light and healthfully, your body will be slimmer. That choice and responsibility lie solely with you.

Just because you desire a certain food, just because you'd love to have a second helping, doesn't mean you have to eat it. You've probably had other self-destructive impulses (such as thinking about having an affair or engaging in illegal or unethical behaviour) that you didn't follow through on. Put eating into that same category, and begin to distinguish between a desire for something and a decision to carry it out. They are entirely different processes. Similarly, a hunger pang does not necessarily signal that it's time to eat. As discussed throughout this book, sometimes what feels like hunger is actually an emotion or stress in disguise. It will also take your stomach approximately one month to become accustomed to a lower-fat diet. Hunger pangs are signals that the body is efficiently using up its calories—a normal sign that the body is doing its job.

Being and staying fit have so many advantages that far outweigh the momentary pleasure of eating a good-tasting meal. Some of the benefits of breaking the Yo-Yo Diet Syndrome cycle include how good it feels:

- ☆ to wear the same size clothing in January as in July;
- ☆ to feel full of energy and zest;
- ☆ to be able to wear a swimsuit out in public and not feel the need to cover up with a bath towel;
- ☆ to feel self-assured that you can accomplish other goals that you set your mind to—in *any* area of your life;

- ☆ to wear shorts even before you have a tan on your legs;
- ☆ to easily and confidently be able to access and follow your intuitive guidance;
- ☆ to enjoy wearing the newest fashions (even the skimpier ones!);
- ☆ to not leave the table feeling stuffed, bloated and out of control;
- ☆ to try on clothes and like the way they look from all angles in the dressing-room mirror;
- ☆ to deal directly with your emotions, instead of stuffing them down with food;
- ☆ to receive admiring glances from others and have others compliment you on your figure;
- ☆ to have more free time, once freed of the obsession with food; and
- ☆ to hear your loved ones compliment you on the way you look.

Beyond all the external extras, the main benefits of breaking the Yo-Yo Diet Syndrome cycle are a tremendous amount of self-respect, confidence and self-love. This is the primary difference between this and your average diet plan. I know because I've been thin many times in the past, but I was never able to enjoy it before because my self-image was so poor. Besides helping me to lose weight and attain healthful fitness, the lessons I learned from the Yo-Yo Diet Syndrome have taught me how to be good to myself. I discovered that I could tailor my life so that I could be happy. That knowledge gave me the courage to take risks so that my real life could match the one I'd always dreamed of. I set occupational, educational, financial, spiritual, physical and emotional goals for myself. I put those goals on my affirmations tape (see Chapter Six) and listened to them daily. And because of my subsequently high level of self-esteem and my belief in myself, I was able to achieve every one of my goals.

I don't want to sound as if I'm boasting, because I'm not. What I want you to know, though, is that I'm no different from you in any way. It wasn't that many years ago when I was 55 pounds overweight, worked at a minimum-wage job that I despised, could barely pay my bills, and was disheartened about my lack of college education—my future seemed as bleak as my life was then.

At that time, I was really down on myself. I felt fat, ugly and unlovable. My only source of comfort seemed to come from tubs of chocolate ice cream. And even though I loathed my bulging thighs that rubbed together as I walked, I didn't know that I had any other option. I didn't know that there was any better way to live. Happiness, I believed, was a myth perpetuated by TV soap operas. Other people were thin and fit. Other people had nice houses and cars. I just didn't think it was in my cards to have a great life.

I thank God that I know differently today! I thank God that I escaped from my self-made hell! And I thank God's intentions for every one of us to have productive, creative, healthful and happy lives.

Now, every day is filled with smiles and feelings of gratitude for all the emotional, spiritual and physical riches that have come my way. Sure, it has meant a lot of work and introspection during the process of getting to know myself. Going to college all those years and working with clients was a struggle at times. And there were moments when I would have done anything to eat some chocolate ice cream.

But I can assure you, as one who has been on both sides of the fence, that the life I lead today—as a fit person who is living a God-given life of love and purpose—tastes a million times better than any scoop of ice cream I've ever had!

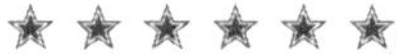

NOTES

(*Editorial Note:* In cases where more than one journal study appears underneath a number, they are arranged in chronological order, with the most recent study appearing first, and the oldest study appearing last.)

CHAPTER 1: THE YO-YO DIET SYNDROME

1. Roberts, C., The effects of stress on food choice, mood and bodyweight in healthy women, *British Nutrition Foundation Nutrition Bulletin*, Vol. 33, 2008. pp. 33–39.

Raikkonen, K., Matthews, K. & Kuller. L., Depressive symptoms and stressful life events predict metabolic syndrome among middle-aged women, *Diabetes Care*, Vol. 30 (4), April 2007. pp. 872–877.

Smith, B., Shelley, B., Leahigh, L. & Vanleit, B., A preliminary study of the effects of a modified mindfulness intervention on binge eating, *Complementary Health Practice Review*, Vol. 11, October 2006, pp. 133.

Brown, M. & Shirley, J., Enhancing women's mood and energy, *The Nurse Practitioner*, Vol. 31 (8), August 2006. pp. 46–53.

Maglione-Garves, C., *Cortisol Connection: Tips on Managing Stress and Weight, Health and Fitness*, Vol. 9 (5), September/October 2005. pp. 20–23.

Gluck, M., Geliebter, A., Hung, J. & Yahav, E., Cortisol, hunger, and desire to binge eat following a cold stress test in obese women with binge eating disorder, *Psychosomatic Medicine*, Vol. 66, 2004. pp. 876–881.

Laporte, L. & Guttman, H., Abusive relationships in families of women with borderline personality disorder, anorexia nervosa and a control group, *The Journal of Nervous and Mental Disease*, Vol. 189 (8), 2001, pp. 522–531.

Ottley, C., Food and mood, *Nursing Standard*, Vol. 15 (2), 27 September 2000, pp. 46-52, 54–55.

Chaouloff, F., Effects of acute physical exercise on central serotonergic systems, *Medicine & Science in Sports & Exercise*, Vol. 29 (1), January 1997. pp. 58–62.

National Health and Nutrition Examination Survey, 1996. Paper presented by Katherine Flegal of the National Center for Health Statistics in Hyattsville, MD, to the North American Association for the Study of Obesity, 1996. Survey of 30,000 subjects conducted from 1991 to 1994.

Xavier, P., The fattening of America, *The Journal of the American Medical Association*, Vol. 272 (3), July 1994, pp. 238–239.

Bray, G., York, B. & DeLany, J., A survey of the opinions of obesity experts on the causes and treatment of obesity, The *American Journal of Clinical Nursing*, Vol 55, 1992. pp. 151S–154S.

2. Raikkonen, K., Matthews, K. & Kuller, L., op. cit.

Smith, B., Shelley, B., Leahigh, L. & Vanleit, B., op.cit.

Janssen, I., Katzmarzyk, P., Boyce, W., Vereecken, C., Mulvihill, C., Roberts, C., Currie, C., Pickett, W., & The Health Behaviour in School-Aged Children Obesity Working Group. Comparison of overweight and obesity prevalence in school-aged youth from 34 countries and their relationships with physical activity and dietary patterns, *Obesity Reviews*, Vol. 6, 2006, pp. 123–132.

Hydock, C., A brief overview of bariatric surgical procedures currently being used to treat the obese patient, *Critical Care Nursing*, Vol. 28 (3), July-September 2005, pp. 217–226.

Nebeling, L., Rogers, C., Berrigan, D., Hursting, S. & Ballard-Barbash, R., Weight cycling and immunocompetence, *Journal of The American Dietetic Association*, Vol. 104 (6), June 2004, pp. 892–894.

Gluck, M., Geliebter, A., Hung, J. & Yahav, E., op.cit.

Vincent, S., Pangrazi, R., Raustorp., Michaud Tomson, L. & Cuddihy, T., Activity levels and body-mass index of children in the United States, Sweden, and Australia, *American College of Sports Medicine*, Vol. 3508, 2003, pp. 1367–1373.

Johnson, J., Spitzer, R. & Williams, J., Health problems, impairment and illnesses associated with bulimia nervosa and binge eating disorder among primary care and obstetric gynaecology patients, *Psychological Medicine*, Vol. 31 (8), November 2001, pp. 1455–1466.

Jeffcoate, W., Obesity is a disease: food for thought, *The Lancet*, Vol. 351, 1998, pp. 903–904.

Jeffrey, R., Does weight cycling present a health risk?, *The American Journal of Clinical Nutrition*, Vol. 63 (suppl), 1996, pp. 452S–455S.

National Task Force on the Prevention and Treatment of Obesity. Weight cycling, The Journal of the American Medical Association, Vol. 272 (15), 19 October 1994, pp. 1196–1202.

Xavier, P., The fattening of America, The *Journal of the American Medical Association*, Vol. 272 (3), July 1994, pp. 238–239.

Prentice, A., Jebb, S., Goldberg, G., Coward, W., Murgatroyd, P., Poppitt, S. & Cole, T., Effects of weight cycling on body composition, *The American Journal of Clinical Nutrition*, Vol. 56, 1992, pp. 209S–216S.

Bray, G., York, B. & DeLany, J., A survey of the opinions of obesity experts on the causes and treatment of obesity, *The American Journal of Clinical Nursing*, Vol 55, 1992. pp. 151S–154S.

3. Roberts, C., The effects of stress on food choice, mood and bodyweight in healthy women, *British Nutrition Foundation Nutrition Bulletin*, Vol. 33, 2008. pp. 33–39.

Mamun, A., Lawlor, D., O'Callaghan, M., Bor, W., Williams, G. & Najman J., Does childhood sexual abuse predict young adult's bmi? a birth cohort study, *Obesity*, Vo. 15 (8), August 2007, pp. 2103–2110.

Smith, B., Shelley, B., Leahigh, L. & Vanleit, B., op.cit.

Rojo, L., Conesa, L., Bermudez, O. & Livianos, L., Influence of stress in the onset of eating disorders: data from a two-stage epidemiologic controlled study, *Psychosomatic Medicine*, Vol. 68 (4), July/August 2006, pp. 628–635.

Maglione-Garves, C., op.cit.

Fontenells, L., An empirical comparison of atypical bulimia nervosa and binge eating disorder, *Brazilian Journal of Medical and Biological Research*, Vol. 38 (11), 2005, pp.1663–1667.

Grilo, C., Masheb., R., Brody, M., Toth, C., Burke-Martindale, C. & Rothschild, B., Childhood maltreatment in extremely obese male and female bariatric surgery candidates, *Obesity Research*, Vol. 13 (1), January 2005, pp. 123–129.

Gluck, M., Geliebter, A., Hung, J. & Yahav, E., op.cit.

Lockwood, R., Lawson, R. & Waller, G., Compulsive features in the eating disorders: a role for trauma?, *The Journal of Nervous and Mental Disease*, Vol. 192 (3), March 2004, pp. 247–249.

Rogge, M., Greenwald, M. & Golden, A., Obesity, stigma, and civilized oppression, *Advances in Nursing Science*, Vol 27 (4), 27 October 2004, pp. 301–315.

Laporte, L. & Guttman, H., abusive relationships in families of women with borderline personality disorder, anorexia nervosa and a control group, *The Journal of Nervous and Mental Disease*, Vol. 189 (8), 2001, pp. 522–531.

Johnson, J., Spitzer, R. & Williams, J., op.cit.

Bulik, C., Prescott, C. & Kendler, K., Features of childhood sexual abuse and the development of psychiatric and substance use disorders, *British Journal of Psychiatry*, Vol. 179, 2001, pp. 444–449.

Toshihiko, N., Matsuyams, M., Kiriike, N., Iketani, T. & Oshima, J., Stress coping strategy in japanese patients with eating disorders: relationship with bulimic and impulsive behaviours, *The Journal of Nervous and Mental Disease*, Vol. 188 (5), May 2000, pp. 280–286.

Wonderlich, S., Crosby, R., Mitchell, J., Roberts, J., Haseltine, B., DeMuth, G. & Thompson, K., Relationship of childhood sexual abuse and eating disturbance in children, journal of the american academy of child and adolescent psychiatry, Vol. 9 (10), October 2000.

Lyons, M., The phenomenon of compulsive overeating in a selected group of professional women, *Journal of Advanced Nursing*, Vol. 27 (6), June 1998, pp. 1158–1164.

Ottley, C., Food and mood, *Nursing Standard*, Vol. 15 (2), 27 September 2000, pp. 46–52, 54–55.

Telch, C.F. & Agras, W.S. (1994). Obesity, binge eating and psychopathology: Are they related? *International Journal of Eating Disorders*, Vol. 15, No. 1, pp. 53–61. Wadden, T.A., et al. (1993).

Bray, G., York, B. & DeLany, J., A survey of the opinions of obesity experts on the causes and treatment of obesity, *The American Journal of Clinical Nursing*, Vol 55, 1992. pp. 151S–154S.

Metabolic, anthropometric, and psychological characteristics of obese binge eaters. *International Journal of Eating Disorders*, Vol. 14, pp. 17–25.

Goldsmith, S.J., et al. (1992). Psychiatric illness in patients presenting for obesity treatment. *International Journal of Eating Disorders,* Vol. 12, No. 1, pp. 63–71.

Marcus, M.D., et al. (1990). Psychiatric disorders among obese binge eaters. *International Journal of Eating Disorders,* Vol. 9, pp. 69–77.

Marcus, M.D., et al. (1988). Obese binge eaters: affect, cognitions, and response to behavioural weight control. *Journal of Consulting and Clinical Psychology*, Vol. 56, pp. 433–439.

4. Rukavina, P. & Li, W., School physical activity interventions: do not forget about obesity bias, *Obesity*, Vol. 9, 2007, pp. 67–76.

Stroch, E., Milsom, V., DeBraganze, N., Lewin, A., Geffken, G. & Silverstein, J., Peer victimization, psychosocial adjustment, and physical activity in overweight and at-risk-for-overweight youth, *Journal of Pediatric Psychology*, Vol. 32 (1), April 2006, pp. 80–89.

Richardson, L., Garrison, M., Drangsholt, M., Mancl, L. & LeResche, L., Association between depressive symptoms and obesity during puberty, *General Hospital Psychiatry*, Vol. 28, 2006, pp. 313–320.

Janssen, I., Craig, W., Boyce, W. & Pickett, W., Associations Between Overweight and Obesity With Bullying Behaviours in School-Aged Children, *Pediatrics,* Vol. 113, 2004, pp. 1187–1194

Rogge, M., Greenwald, M. & Golden, A., op.cit.

Kuehnel, R.H. & Wadden, T.A. (1994). Binge eating disorder, weight cycling, and psychopathology. *International Journal of Eating Disorders,* Vol. 15, No. 4, pp. 321–329.

deZwaan, M., et al. (1994). Eating related and general psychopathology in obese females with binge eating disorder. *International Journal of Eating Disorders,* Vol. 15, No. 1, pp. 43–52.

5. Roberts, C., The effects of stress on food choice, mood and bodyweight in healthy women, *British Nutrition Foundation Nutrition Bulletin*, Vol. 33, 2008. pp. 33–39.

Dalton, S., Focus on obesity and weight management – obesity trends past, present and future, *Topics in Clinical Nutrition*, Vol. 21 (2), 2006, pp. 76–94.

Hydock, C., A brief overview of bariatric surgical procedures currently being used to treat the obese patient, *Critical Care Nursing*, Vol. 28 (3), July-September 2005, pp. 217–226.

Walton, K., Schneider, R. & Nidich, S., Review of controlled research on the transcendental meditation program and cardiovascular disease risk factors, morbidity, and mortality, *Cardiology in Review*, Vol. 12 (5), September/October 2004, pp. 262–266.

Canter, P., The therapeutic effects of meditation, *BMJ*, Vol. 326, 2003, pp. 1049–1050.

Bonadonna, R., Meditation's impact on chronic illness, *Holistic Nurse Practitioner*, Vol. 17 (6), 2003, pp. 309–319.

Ottley, C., Food and mood, *Nursing Standard*, Vol. 15 (2), 27 September 2000, pp. 46–52, 54–55.

Peden, A., Hall, L., Rayens, M. & Beebe, L., Reducing negative thinking and depressive symptoms in college women, *Journal of Nursing Scholarship*, Vol. 32 (2), 2000, pp. 145–151

Vickers, A. & Zollman, C., ABC of complementary medicine: hypnosis and relaxation therapies, *BMJ*, Vol. 319, 1999, pp. 1346–1349.

Jeffrey, R., op.cit.

National Task Force on the Prevention and Treatment of Obesity., Weight cycling, *The Journal of the American Medical Association*, Vol. 272 (15), 19 October 1994, pp. 1196–1202

Foreyt, J.P. (1995). Psychological correlates of weight fluctuation. *International Journal of Eating Disorders,* Vol. 17, No. 3, pp. 263–275.

Kuhnel, R.H. (1994), op.cit.

Grilo, C.M., et al. (1994). Binge eating antecedents in normal-weight non-purging females: Is there consistency? *International Journal of Eating Disorders,* Vol. 16, No.3, pp. 239–249.

Lowe, M. (1993). The effects of dieting on eating behaviour: A three-factor model. *Psychological Bulletin*, Vol. 114, pp. 100–121.

6. Beaver, J., Lawrence, A., van Ditzhuijzen, J., Davis, M., Woods, A. & Calder, A., Individual differences in reward drive predict neural responses to images of food, *The Journal of Neuroscience*, Vol. 26 (19), 10 May 2006, pp. 5160–5166.

Ledikwe, J., Ello-Martin, J. & Rolls, B., Portion sizes and the obesity epidemic, *Journal of Nutrition*, Vol. 135, 2005, pp. 905–909.

Levitsky, D. & Youn, T., The more food young adults are served, the more they overeat, *The Journal of Nutrition*, Vol. 134, 2004, pp. 2546–2549.

Jeffery, R. & French, S., Epidemic Obesity in the United States: Are Fast Foods and Television Viewing Contributing?, *American Journal of Public Health*, Vol. 88 (2) February 1998, pp. 277–280

DeJong, W. (1980) The stigma of obesity: The consequences of naïve assumptions concerning the causes of physical deviance. *Journal of Health and Social Behaviour*, Vol. 21, pp. 75–87.

McLean, R.A. & Moon, M. (1980). Health, obesity and earnings. *American Journal of Public Health*, Vol. 70, pp. 1006–1009.

Larkin, J.C. & Pines, H.A. (1979). No fat persons need apply: Experimental studies of the overweight sterotype and hiring preference.

Canning, H. & Mayer, J. (1966). Obesity—its possible effect on college acceptance. *New England Journal of Medicine*, Vol. 275, pp. 1172–1174.

Richardson, S.A., et al. (1961). Cultural uniformity in reaction to physical disabilities. *American Sociological Review*, Vol. 90, pp. 44–54.

CHAPTER 2: SPIRITUAL SOLUTIONS FOR THE YO-YO DIET SYNDROME

1. Marwick, C. (1995). Should physicians prescribe prayer for health? Spiritual aspects of well-being considered. *Journal of the American Medical Association*, Vol. 273, No. 20, pp. 1561–1562.

Wirth, D.P. (1995). The significance of belief and expectancy within the spiritual healing encounter. *Social Science Medicine*, Vol. *41*, 2, pp. 249–260.

2. Foundation for Inner Peace (1975). *A Course in Miracles.* Glen Ellen, California.

3. Rodin, J., et al. (1985). Effects of insulin and glucose on feeding behaviour. *Metabolism*, Vol. 34, pp. 826–831.

Rodin, J. (1980). The externality theory today. In: Stunkard, A.J. (Ed.), *Obesity*. Philadelphia: Saunders.

Watson, R. (1980). Psychological influences on eating behaviour. In: Turner, M. (Ed.), *Nutrition and Lifestyles*, pp. 43–52. London: Applied Science Publishers, Ltd.

CHAPTER 7: THE STRESS EATERS

1. Brown, M. & Shirley, J., Enhancing women's mood and energy, *The Nurse Practitioner*, Vol. 31 (8), August 2006. pp. 46–53.

Dalton, S., Focus on obesity and weight management–obesity trends past, present and future, *Topics in Clinical Nutrition*, Vol. 21 (2), 2006, pp. 76–94.

Doraiswamy, P. & Xiong, G., Longevity and optimal health, *Annals of the New York Academy of Sciences*, December 2006, ID. 1393.002.

Warburton, D., Nicol, C. & Bredin, S., Health benefits of physical activity: the evidence, *CMAJ*, Vol. 174 (6), 14 March 2006, pp. 801–809.

Daley, A., Copeland, R., Wright, N., Roalfe, A. & Wales, J., Exercise therapy as a treatment for psychopathologic conditions in obese and morbidly obese adolescents: a randomized, controlled trial, *Pediatrics*, Vol. 118, 2006, pp. 2126–2134.

Walton, K., Schneider, R. & Nidich, S., Review of controlled research on the transcendental meditation program and cardiovascular disease risk factors, morbidity, and mortality, *Cardiology in Review*, Vol. 12 (5), September/October 2004, pp. 262–266.

Canter, P., The therapeutic effects of meditation, *BMJ*, Vol. 326, 2003, pp. 1049–1050.

Bonadonna, R., Meditation's impact on chronic illness, *Holistic Nurse Practitioner*, Vol. 17 (6), 2003, pp. 309–319.

Ottley, C., Food and mood, *Nursing Standard*, Vol. 15 (2), 27 September 2000, pp. 46–52, 54–55.

Peden, A., Hall, L., Rayens, M. & Beebe, L., Reducing negative thinking and depressive symptoms in college women, *Journal of Nursing Scholarship*, Vol. 32 (2), 2000, pp. 145–151.

Vickers, A. & Zollman, C., ABC of complementary medicine: hypnosis and relaxation therapies, *BMJ*, Vol. 319, 1999, pp. 1346–1349.

Chaouloff, F., Effects of acute physical exercise on central serotonergic systems, *Medicine & Science in Sports & Exercise*, Vol. 29 (1), January 1997. pp. 58–62.

King, N., Tremblay, A. & Blundell, J., Effects of exercise on appetite control implications for balance, *Medicine and Science in Sports & Exercise*, Vol 29 (8), August 1997, pp. 1076–1089.

Sharma, H.S., et al. (1991). Increased blood-brain barrier permeability following acute short-term swimming exercise in conscious normotensive young rats. *Neuroscience Research,* Vol. 10, No. 3, pp. 211–221.

Naesh, O., et al. (1990). Post-exercise platelet activation: aggregation and release in relation to dynamic exercise. *Clinical Physiology,* Vol. 10, No. 3, pp. 221–230.

Blomstrand, E., et al. (1989). Effect of sustained exercise on plasma amino acid concentrations and on 5-hydroxytrptamine metabolism in six different brain regions in the rat. *Acta Physiological Scandia,*Vol. 136, pp. 473–481.

Chaouloff, F. (1989). Physical exercise and brain monoamines: a review. *Acta Physiological Scandia,* Vol. 137, pp. 1–13.

Chaouloff, F. (1989). Physical exercise: evidence for differential consequences of tryptophan on 5-HT synthesis and metabolism in central serotonergic cell bodies and terminals. *Journal of Neural Transmission,* Vol. 78, pp. 121–130.

2. Roberts, C., op.cit.

Brown, M. & Shirley, J., op.cit.

Smith, B., Shelley, B., Leahigh, L. & Vanleit, B., op.cit.

Maglione-Garves, C., Cortisol connection: tips on managing stress and weight, *Health and Fitness*, Vol. 9 (5), September/October 2005. pp. 20–23.

Gluck, M., Geliebter, A., Hung, J. & Yahav, E., op.cit.

Ottley, C., op.cit.

Bray, G., York, B. & DeLany, J., A survey of the opinions of obesity experts on the causes and treatment of obesity, The *American Journal of Clinical Nursing*, Vol 55, 1992. pp. 151S–154S.

Walton, K. G., et al. (1994). A neuroendocrine mechanism for the reduction of drug use and addictions by Trancendental Meditation. *Alcoholism Treatment Quarterly*, Vol. 11, Nos. 1-2, pp. 89–117.

Alexander, C.N., et al. (1989). Transcendental meditation, mindfulness, and longevity: An experimental study with the elderly. *Journal of Personality and Social Psychology,* Vol. 57, No. 6, pp. 950–964.

Morse, D.R. (1988) Aging: causes and control. *International Journal of Psychosomatics,* Vol. 34, Nos. 1-4, pp. 12–42.

CHAPTER 8: THE SNOWBALL EFFECT EATERS

1. Ledikwe, J., Ello-Martin, J. & Rolls, B., Portion sizes and the obesity epidemic, *Journal of Nutrition,* Vol. 135, 2005, pp. 905–909.

Levitsky, D. & Youn, T., The more food young adults are served, the more they overeat,, *The Journal of Nutrition,* Vol. 134, 2004, pp. 2546–2549.

Beaver, J., Lawrence, A., van Ditzhuijzen, J., Davis, M., Woods, A. & Calder, A., Individual differences in reward drive predict neural responses to images of food, *The Journal of Neuroscience,* Vol. 26 (19), 10 May 2006, pp. 5160–5166.

Duffey, K., Gordon-Larsen, P., Jacobs, D., Williams, O. & Popkin, B., Differential associations of fast food and restaurant food consumption with 3-y change in body-mass index: the coronary artery risk development in young adults study, *American Journal of Clinical Nutrition,* Vol. 85, 2007, pp. 201–208.

Cummings, D., Frayo, R., Marmonier, C., Aubert, R. & Chapelot, D., Plasma ghrelin levels and hunger scores in humans initiating meals voluntarily without time- and food-related cues, *American Journal Physiology Endocrinology and Metabolism,* Vol. 287, 2004, pp. E297–E304.

Jeffcoate, W., op.cit.

Jeffery, R. & French, S., op.cit.

LeMagnen, J. (1985). *Hunger.* Cambridge, England: Cambridge University Press.

Rolls, B.J., et al. (1981). Variety in a meal enhances food intake in man. *Physiology and Behaviour,* Vol. 26, pp. 215–221.

Rolls, B., et al. (1980). Appetite and obesity: Influences of sensory stimuli and external cues. In: Turner, M. (Ed.), *Nutrition and Lifestyles,* pp. 11–19. Essex, England: Applied Science Publishers.

CHAPTER 9: PRACTICAL GUIDANCE ON EATING RIGHT

1. Koella, W.P. (1988). Serotonin and sleep. In: *Neuronal Serotonin*, Osborne, N.N. & Hamon, M. (Eds.). New York: John Wiley and Sons.

Henriksen, S., et al. (1974). The role of serotonin in the regulation of a phasic event of rapid eye movement sleep: The pontogeniculo-occipital wave. *Advances in Biochemical Psychopharmacology*, Vol. 11, pp. 169–179.

Wyatt, R.J. (1974). Ventricular fluid 5-hydroxyindoleacetic acid concentrations during human sleep. *Advances in Biochemical Psychopharmacology*, Vol. 11, pp. 193–197.

2. Penev, P., Sleep deprivation and energy metabolism: to sleep, perchance to eat?, endocrinology, *Diabetes & Obesity*, Vol. 14, 2007, pp. 374–381.

Lamberg, L., Rx for Obesity: Eat less, exercise more, and – maybe – get more sleep, *Journal of The American Medical Association*, Vol. 295 (20), 24/31 May 2006, pp. 2341–2344.

Lean, M. & Hankey, C., Aspartame and its effects on health, *BMJ*, vol. 329, 2 October 2004, pp. 755–756.

Rolls, B., Effects of intense sweeteners on hunger, food intake, and body weight: a review, *American Journal of Clinical Nutrition*, Vol. 53, 1991, pp. 872–878.

Anderson, G.H. & Leiter, L.A. (1988). Effects of aspartame and phenylalanine on meal-time food intake of humans. *Appetite*, Vol. 11 (Supp.), pp. 48–53.

Fernstrom, J.D. (1988). Carbohydrate ingestion and brain serotonin synthesis: Relevance to a putative control loop for regulating carbohydrate ingestion, and effects of aspartame consumption. *Appetite*, Vol. 11 (Supp.), pp. 35–41.

Yokogoshi, H., Roberts, C., Caballero, B. & Wurtman, R., Effects of aspartame and glucose administration on brain and plasma levels of large neutral amino acids and brain 5-hydroxyindoles, *The American Journal of Clinical Nutrition*, Vol. 40, July 1984, pp. 1–7.

3. Mosnaim, A.D. & Wolf, M.E. (Eds.) (1978). *Noncatechoic Phenylethylamines, Part 1: Phenylethylamine: Biological Mechanisms and Clinical Aspects.* New York: Marcel Dekker, Inc.

McKean, C.M. (1972). The effects of high phenylalanine concentrations on serotonin and catecholamine metabolism in the human brain. *Brain Research,* Vol. 47, pp. 469–476.

4. Anderson, G.H. (1988). Op. cit.

Porikos, K.P. & Koopmans, H.S. (1988). The effects of non-nutritive sweeteners on body weight in rats. *Appetite,* Vol. 11 (Supp.), pp. 12–15.

Brala, P.M. & Hagen, R.L. (1983). Effects of sweetness perception and caloric value of a preload on short-term intake. *Physiology and Behaviour,* Vol. 30, pp. 1–9.

5. Powell, A. (2005). The Royal College of Psychiatrists The Contribution of Spirit Release Therapy to Mental Health, http://www.rcpsych.ac.uk/PDF/AndrewPowell34TheContributionSpirit.pdf (Accessed 20 March 2008).

Sanderson, A. (2003). The Royal College of Psychiatrists, Spirit Release Therapy: What Is It and What Can It Achieve: A Clinical Presentation of Therapist and Patient Perspectives.

http://www.rcpsych.ac.uk/PDF/Sanderson_01_jun_03.pdf (Accessed 20 March 2008).

Sanderson, A. (1998). Spirit Release Foundation Spirit Releasement Therapy.

http://www.spiritrelease.com/cases/clara.htm (Accessed 20 March 2008).

Baldwin, W. (1992) Spirit Releasement Therapy: A Technique-Manual, Second Edition. Terra Alta, WV: Headline Books, Inc.

CHAPTER 10: EXERCISE FOR THE BODY, MIND AND SOUL

1. Sharma, H.S., et al. (1991). Increased blood–brain barrier permeability following acute short-term swimming exercise in conscious normotensive young rats. *Neuroscience Research,* Vol. 10, No. 3, pp. 211–221.

Naesh, O., et al. (1990). Post-exercise platelet activation: Aggregation and release in relation to dynamic exercise. *Clinical Physiology*, Vol. 10, No. 3, pp. 221–230.

Blomstrand, E., et al. (1989). Effect of sustained exercise on plasma amino acid concentrations and on 5-hydroxytryptamine metabolism in six different rat regions in the rat. *Acta Physiological Scandia*, Vol. 136, pp. 473–481.

Chaouloff, F. (1989). Physical exercise and brain monoamines: A review. *Acta Physiological Scandia*, Vol. 137, pp. 1–13.

Chaouloff, F. (1989). Physical exercise: Evidence for differential consequences of tryptophan on 5-HT synthesis and metabolism in central serotonergic cell bodies and terminals. *Journal of Neural Transmission*, Vol. 78, pp. 121–130.

2. Brown, M. & Shirley, J., Enhancing women's mood and energy, *The Nurse Practitioner*, Vol. 31 (8), August 2006. pp. 46–53.

Warburton, D., Nicol, C. & Bredin, S., Health benefits of physical activity: the evidence, *CMAJ*, Vol. 174 (6), 14 March 2006, pp. 801–809.

Daley, A., Copeland, R., Wright, N., Roalfe, A. & Wales, J., Exercise therapy as a treatment for psychopathologic conditions in obese and morbidly obese adolescents: a randomized, controlled trial, *Pediatrics*, Vol. 118, 2006, pp. 2126–2134.

Maglione-Garves, C., Cortisol connection: tips on managing stress and weight, *Health and Fitness*, Vol. 9 (5), September/October 2005. pp. 20–23.

Scott, S., Combating depression with exercise, ACSM's *Health & Fitness Journal*, Vol. 9 (4) July/August 2005, pp. 31–33.

Ottley, C., Food and mood, *Nursing Standard*, Vol. 15 (2), 27 September 2000, pp. 46–52, 54–55.

Chaouloff, F., Effects of acute physical exercise on central serotonergic systems, *Medicine & Science in Sports & Exercise*, Vol. 29 (1), January 1997. pp. 58–62.

Dyer, J.B. & Crouch, J.G. (1988). Effects of running and other activities on moods. *Perceptual and Motor Skills*, Vol. 67, pp. 43–50.

Labbe, E.E., et al. (1988). Effects of consistent aerobic exercise on the psychological functioning of women. *Perceptual and Motor Skills*, Vol. 67, pp. 919–925.

Netz, Y., et al. (1988). Pattern of psychological fitness as related to pattern of physical fitness among older adults. *Perceptual and Motor Skills,* Vol. 67, pp. 647–655.

McCann, I.L. & Holmes, D.S. (1984). Influence of aerobic exercise on depression. *Journal of Personality and Social Psychology,* Vol. 46, No. 5, pp. 1142–1147.

3. Bolton, B. & Renfrow, N.E. (1979). Personality characteristics associated with aerobic exercise in adult females. *Journal of Personality and Assessment.* Vol. 43, No. 5, pp. 504–508.

SELF-HELP RESOURCES

The following list of resources can be used to access information on a variety of issues. The addresses and telephone numbers listed are for the national headquarters; look in your local Yellow Pages under "Community Services" for resources closer to your area.

AIDS

Terence Higgins Trust
0845 12 21 200
www.tht.org.uk

National AIDS Trust
New City Cloisters
196 Old Street
London EC1V 9F4
020 7814 6767
www.nat.org.uk

ALCOHOL ABUSE

Alcohol Concern
020 7264 0510
www.alcoholconcern.org.uk

Alcoholics Anonymous
0845 769 7555 (helpline)
www.alcoholics-anonymous.org.uk

Drinkline
0800 917 8282

Al-Anon Family Groups UK & Eire
61 Great Dover Street
London
SE1 4YF
Tel: 020 7403 0888
www.al-anonuk.org.uk

ALZHEIMER'S DISEASE

Alzheimer's Society
0845 300 0336 (helpline)
www.alzheimers.org.uk

CANCER

CancerHelp UK
020 7061 8355, or freephone 0808 800 4040
www.cancerhelp.org.uk

CHILDREN'S ISSUES

Child Molestation

Childline
Freepost NATN1111,
London E1 6BR
0800 1111 (helpline)
0800 400 222 (textphone service)
www.childline.org.uk

National Society for the Prevention of Cruelty to Children (NSPCC)
Weston House
42 Curtains Road
London EC2A 3NH
020 7825 2500 (administration)
0808 800 5000 (helpline)

Crisis Intervention

Barnardo's
Tanner's Lane
Barkingside
Ilford IG6 1QG
020 8550 8822
www.barnardos.org.uk

Childline
Royal Mail Building
2nd Floor
Studd Street
London N1 OQW
0800 1111 (helpline)
0800 400 222 (textphone service)
www.childline.org.uk

Missing Children

Missing People (Formerly National Missing Persons Helpline)
0500 700 700
www.missingpeople.org

UK Missing and Exploited Children
http://uk.missingkids.com

Children with Serious Illnesses (fulfilling wishes):

Make-a-Wish Foundation UK
01276 405060
www.make-a-wish.org.uk

Starlight Foundation
11-15 Emerald Street
London WC1N 3QL
020 7430 1642
www.starlight.org.uk

CO-DEPENDENCY
DEATH/GRIEVING/SUICIDE

Cruse Bereavement Care
www.crusebereavementcare.org.uk
0844 477 9400

The Compassionate Friends – help for bereaved parents
53 North Street
Bristol BS3 1EN
0845 123 2304 (helpline)
0845 120 3785 (administration)
www.tcf.org.uk

Winston's Wish – help for bereaved children
The Clara Burgess Centre
Gloucestershire Royal Hospital
Great Western Road
Gloucester GL1 3NN
0845 20 30 40 5 (helpline)
www.winstonswish.org.uk

DEBTS

National Debt Helpline
0808 808 4000
www.nationaldebtline.co.uk

DIABETES

Diabetes UK
10 Parkway
London NW1 7AA
020 7424 1000
www.diabetesuk.org

DOMESTIC VIOLENCE

Women's Aid
0808 2000 247 (helpline)
www.womensaid.org.uk

DRUG ABUSE

Frank
0800 776600 (helpline)
0800 9178765 (textphone)
www.talktofrank.com

The Centre for Recovery Cyswllt Ceredigion Contact
49 North Parade
Ceredigion SY23 2JN
01970 626470
www.recovery.org.uk

Narcotics Anonymous—UK Region
0800 373 3366
www.ukna.org

EATING DISORDERS

beat (formerly Eating Disorders Association)
103 Prince of Wales Road
Norwich NR1 1DW
0845 634 1414 (adults)
0845 634 7650 (youth)
www.edauk.com/www.b-eat.co.uk

GAMBLING

Gamblers Anonymous UK
PO Box 5382 London W1A 6SA
020 7384 3040 (helpline)
www.gamblersanonymous.org.uk

HEALTH ISSUES

National Health Service (NHS) Direct
0845 4647 (24-hour nurse advice line)
www.nhsdirect.nhs.uk

HOUSING RESOURCES

The Abbeyfield Society
(for elderly people)
The Abbeyfield House
53 Victoria St.
St Albans
Herts AL1 3UW
01727 857536
www.abbeyfield.com

Centrepoint (for young people)
0845 466 3400
www.centrepoint.org.uk

Shelterline
0808 800 4444
www.shelter.org.uk

IMPOTENCE

Sexual Dysfunction Association
Suite 301
Emblem House
London Bridge Hospital
27 Tooley Street
London SE1 2PR
0870 7743571
www.sda.net

MENTAL HEALTH

Mind (The National Association for Mental Health)
15-19 Broadway
London E15 4BQ
0870 7660163
www.mind.org.uk

SANE
1st Floor
Cityside House
40 Adler Street
London E1 1EE
020 7375 1002
0845 767 8000 (SANEline, open noon–2 a.m.)
www.sane.org.uk

PET BEREAVEMENT

Animal Samaritans
52 Verdant Lane
London SE3 1LF
020 8303 1859
www.animalsamaritans.org.uk/bereave.htm

RAPE/SEXUAL ISSUES

Rape Crisis Federation of Wales and England
7 Mansfield Rd.
Nottingham NG1 3FB
0115 934 8474
www.rapecrisis.co.uk

Rape and Sexual Abuse Counselling
01962 848018 (administration)
01962 848024 (helpline for women)
01962 848027 (helpline for men)
http://rasac.org.uk

SMOKING

Quit
0800 00 22 00
www.quit.org.uk

STRESS REDUCTION

International Stress Management Association
P.O. Box 348
Waltham Cross EN8 8ZL
07000 780430
www.isma.org.uk

TEEN HELP

www.teenhelp.org
www.teenissues.co.uk

INDEX

ABOUT THE AUTHOR

Doreen Virtue, PhD, holds three university degrees in counselling psychology and is a fourth-generation metaphysician specializing in helping her clients identify and manifest true purpose and desire. She is the best-selling author of many books, including *Losing Your Pounds of Pain, Solomon's Angels*, and *How to Hear Your Angels*, and appears often on radio and television shows.

NOTES

NOTES

We hope you enjoyed this Hay House book.
If you would like to receive a free catalogue featuring additional Hay House books and products, or if you would like information about the Hay Foundation, please contact:

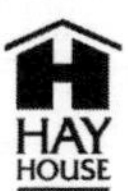

Hay House UK Ltd
292B Kensal Rd • London W10 5BE
Tel: (44) 20 8962 1230; Fax: (44) 20 8962 1239
www.hayhouse.co.uk

***

Published and distributed in the United States of America by:
Hay House, Inc. • PO Box 5100 • Carlsbad, CA 92018-5100
Tel.: (1) 760 431 7695 or (1) 800 654 5126;
Fax: (1) 760 431 6948 or (1) 800 650 5115
www.hayhouse.com

Published and distributed in Australia by:
Hay House Australia Ltd • 18/36 Ralph St • Alexandria NSW 2015
Tel.: (61) 2 9669 4299; Fax: (61) 2 9669 4144
www.hayhouse.com.au

Published and distributed in the Republic of South Africa by:
Hay House SA (Pty) Ltd • PO Box 990 • Witkoppen 2068
Tel./Fax: (27) 11 467 8904 • www.hayhouse.co.za

Published and distributed in India by:
Hay House Publishers India • Muskaan Complex • Plot No.3
B-2 • Vasant Kunj • New Delhi – 110 070.
Tel.: (91) 11 41761620; Fax: (91) 11 41761630.
www.hayhouse.co.in

Distributed in Canada by:
Raincoast • 9050 Shaughnessy St • Vancouver, BC V6P 6E5
Tel.: (1) 604 323 7100; Fax: (1) 604 323 2600

***